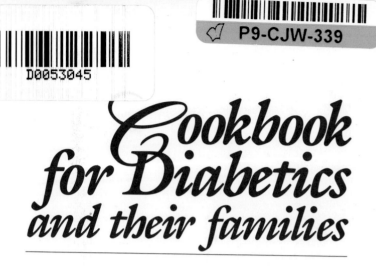

Cookbook for Diabetics and their families

Foreword by James A. Pittman, Jr., M.D.

Dean, University of Alabama School of Medicine
University of Alabama in Birmingham

Developed by Registered Dietitians of the General
Clinical Research Center and the Department of
Dietetics of the University of Alabama Hospitals at
the University of Alabama in Birmingham.

Oxmoor
House®

Library of Congress Catalog Number: 84-60289
ISBN: 0-8487-0633-1

Manufactured in the United States of America
Sixth Printing 1986

Production Editor: Joan Denman
Editorial Assistant: Patty E. Howdon
Designer: Faith Nance
Illustrator: Barbara Shores

Editor: Betty Darnell, M.S., R.D.
  General Clinical Research Center

Cover:
Jim Bathie, Photographer
Sara Jane Ball, Food Stylist

Cover (clockwise from front): Creole Chicken on
rice (page 117), "Creamy" Sliced Cucumber Salad
(page 133), Sautéed Zucchini (page 162), Biscuits
(page 44), Brandied Oranges (page 57).

CONTENTS

iv

ACKNOWLEDGEMENTS

We gratefully acknowledge the contributions several people have made in the development of the *Cookbook for Diabetics and their families*. Special thanks to Mandy Berry, Laura Moore, and Deborah Ramsey, Research Cooks from the General Clinical Research Center, who prepared all recipes; to Karen Anderson, M.S., R.D., Janice Allen, R.D., Vesta Johnson, R.D., Lynn Epps, R.D., and Lori White, R.D., for their contributions; to Ann Harrell, Assistant to the Director of the G.C.R.C., Sandra Dillon, R.D., Associate Director of the Department of Dietetics, and Linda Godfrey, M.S., R.D., Chief Clinical Dietitian, Department of Dietetics, for their encouragement and support.

Many thanks to the Dietetic Interns from the Dietetic Internship Program, Department of Nutrition Sciences, University of Alabama in Birmingham; Registered Dietitians of the Department of Dietetics; and the Staff of the G.C.R.C. for their contributions.

Also, a special thank you to the patients with diabetes and their families whose requests for recipes inspired this cookbook and who offered suggestions for its contents.

Betty Darnell, M.S., R.D.
General Clinical Research Center

FOREWORD

A proper diet is a major foundation of good health—one of the four pillars of health—and that is what this book is about. Eating is not only essential to life, but can also be one of life's most pleasurable activities. The *Cookbook for Diabetics and their families* was developed to make eating enjoyable and interesting, as well as healthful for the entire family.

Dr. Tinsley Harrison, founding Chairman of Medicine at the University of Alabama in Birmingham, at Dallas, and at Winston-Salem's Bowman Gray medical schools, now memorialized in his book *Harrison's Principles of Internal Medicine,* used to say that the diagnosis of a chronic disease can be the first step to living a long and happy life. The implication was that only then does one become sufficiently motivated to give proper attention to his own health care.

"Proper attention to one's own health care" means attending to the Four Pillars of Self Care in Health: Rest, Exercise, Diet and a Tranquil outlook. All four pillars are generally neglected, particularly in affluent industrialized nations and particularly by young people.

So when someone in the family is found to have diabetes mellitus, the whole family can profit by greater attention to the four pillars of health, especially the diet; and this book can be of great help in making a pleasure out of a necessity.

The registered dietitians of the UAB General Clinical Research Center and the Department of Dietetics, University of Alabama Hospitals, are to be congratulated on this fine practical guide to healthy eating. They are experts with a long and successful reputation for the development, planning, and preparation of such meals, and now their expertise is available for all to share.

Good eating, and long life!

James A. Pittman, Jr., M.D.,
Dean, University of Alabama School of Medicine, UAB

INTRODUCTION

Proper nutrition is the foundation of good health and is essential for individuals with diabetes as well as those without it. Those people with diabetes mellitus cannot store and use glucose (blood sugar) effectively. For good blood glucose control, people with diabetes must follow a well-planned diet, avoiding some foods, limiting others, and spacing intake of food. In some instances, diabetes may be managed by diet control alone. In other cases, for those requiring oral hypoglycemic agents or insulin, glucose control is usually better when the individual follows a proper diet.

Our patients with diabetes mellitus and others who use calorie-controlled recipes have expressed a desire to combine their own dietary requirements with those for their families. This recipe collection has been carefully prepared to respond to this need. The recipes in this book can be enjoyed by everyone in the family.

A significant feature of this book is that the recipes are lower in calories than those in the average cookbook. Sugar substitutes and other reduced-calorie ingredients have been used, resulting in a lower caloric content which makes the foods ideal for use by individuals with diabetes as well as the weight-conscious. Most recipes yield average family-size servings with Diabetic Exchanges given so they may be incorporated into the diabetic's meal plan. This book also provides information on basic nutrition for the family plus general information for people with diabetes.

The *Cookbook for Diabetics and their families* was developed jointly by the Registered Dietitians of the General Clinical Research Center and the Department of Dietetics of the University of Alabama Hospitals at the University of Alabama in Birmingham. The recipes were tested and evaluated in the General Clinical Research Center kitchen.

Our goal is to assist you in planning menus that will help the diabetic in your family follow a long term diet and, at the same time, provide nutritional and enjoyable meals for the whole family.

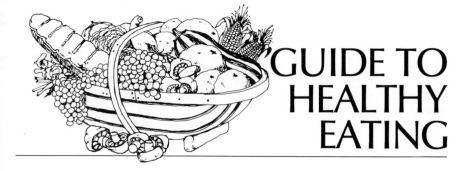

GUIDE TO
HEALTHY
EATING

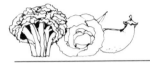

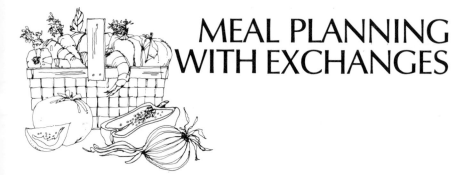

MEAL PLANNING WITH EXCHANGES

Planning meals for a family that includes a diabetic is not difficult when it is realized that a person with diabetes needs the same nutrients as the rest of the family. An overview of these nutrients and their use in the body is discussed in the following pages.

Diabetics do not need to eat "special" foods. The basic guidelines for a diabetic diet are similar to guidelines recommended for everyone to maintain good health. In a typical diabetic meal plan, carbohydrates are provided in controlled amounts and at consistent levels during the day to better regulate blood glucose, and fats are used sparingly because they are high in calories. The individual meal plan for the diabetic, worked out by a registered dietitian (R.D.), reflects these controls and is designed to be used with the nationally accepted Exchange Lists for Meal Planning reprinted here.

The use of the Exchange Lists is a necessity for the person on a controlled diet, but the Lists are also a valuable aid in planning meals for the rest of the family. One important guideline of good health is to eat a variety of foods because no single food or food group contains all the necessary nutrients. The Exchange Lists provide this variety.

This chapter also covers diabetic meal planning for special circumstances, foods appropriate for sick days, and tips on selecting the right foods when eating away from home.

BASIC NUTRITION FOR THE DIABETIC AND FAMILY

Nutrition deals with the food we eat and the use of this food in the body. The basic functions of nutrients are to provide energy; build, maintain, repair, and replace body tissues; and regulate body processes. Foods contain various nutrients that are needed for these complex body functions. We all need the same nutrients each day but in varying amounts based on our sex, size, age, activity, and state of health. The main classes of basic nutrients are carbohydrates, fats, proteins, minerals, vitamins, and water. For additional information regarding the major functions and food sources of these nutrients, refer to page 176.

CARBOHYDRATES

Carbohydrates are important as energy sources, supplying approximately 45% to 50% of the energy in a typical diet. Simple carbohydrates (mono- and disaccharides) are sugars which occur naturally in fruits, milk, some vegetables, and honey.

Refined and processed products such as syrups and brown and white table sugar contain primarily carbohydrates. Diabetics and others watching their weight should avoid these concentrated carbohydrates by reading labels to check for these as added ingredients.

Complex carbohydrates (polysaccharides) are starches and are found in breads, cereals, legumes, and some vegetables. Some complex carbohydrates such as cellulose are important since they add bulk or fiber to the diet. Many research studies have indicated that adding fiber to the diabetic's diet aids in blood glucose control.

FATS

Fats, the most concentrated sources of energy, provide 9 calories per gram and are important carriers of the fat-soluble vitamins A, D, E, and K. Fats contain the essential fatty acids that are needed for body growth.

Excessive intakes of fat are stored in the body as fat tissue. Some stores are important for insulating the body and for cushioning vital organs to protect them from injury. Excessive stores of fat are undesirable and result in overweight or obesity.

Fats are found in many animal foods and some plants. Visible fats include butter, margarine, oils, and fatty deposits on meat; invisible "hidden" fats include marbling of fat within the muscle of meat, cream in milk and cheese, also nuts, chocolate, butter, and other fats or oils in desserts.

There are three types of fatty acids in foods: saturated, monounsaturated, and polyunsaturated. Saturated fats are generally solid at room temperature. Sources are animal products such as meat fat, whole milk, and butter. Also, there is some in coconut oil, cocoa butter (chocolate), and those vegetable margarines and shortenings that have been hydrogenated. Unsaturated fatty acids are generally those that are liquid at room temperature and are found in plant sources such as safflower, corn, soybean, and cottonseed oils.

Research studies have indicated that saturated fats increase blood cholesterol and polyunsaturated fats tend to lower blood cholesterol levels. Cholesterol, a fatty substance found in animal fats, is needed in the body but can be manufactured by the body. Studies have suggested that a high level of blood cholesterol is associated with an increased risk of heart disease. Significant sources of cholesterol are egg yolk, fats in meats, and organ meats.

Fat added to foods will greatly increase their caloric value. To reduce caloric value of any food, limit the fat that is added.

PROTEINS

Proteins are required for growth, maintenance, and repair of body tissues; for manufacture of protein-containing compounds such as hormones, antibodies, and enzymes; and for regulation of fluid balance in cells. If the diet does not contain enough fat and carbohydrate for energy, protein will be used.

Proteins are made up of amino acids. There are 22 amino acids, 9 of which are essential meaning they must be included in the diet to maintain life and promote growth. Proteins are classified according to their amino acid content. "Complete" proteins contain all of the essential amino acids. "Incomplete" proteins contain an inadequate amount of one or more of the essential amino acids.

Proteins found in animal foods, with the exception of gelatin, are complete. Plant proteins are found in legumes, corn, rice, wheat, and other cereals. The plant proteins are "incomplete;" however, legumes (soybeans, lentils, navy beans, pinto beans, peas, red beans, black-eyed peas) are good sources of protein and contribute to the total intake of protein. If eaten in combination, plant proteins will complement each other to provide protein of good quality.

MINERALS

Minerals are inorganic elements that do not provide energy but are necessary for the proper utilization of the energy nutrients: carbohydrates, fats, and proteins.

Macrominerals are those found in the body in greatest quantity, namely, calcium, iron, phosphorus, potassium, sulfur, sodium, chloride, and magnesium. Microminerals are those found in the body in lesser quantity; they are known as trace elements and include zinc, selenium, manganese, copper, iodine, molybdenum, cobalt, and fluorine.

Minerals perform several essential functions in the body: control water balance; regulate acid-base balance; are constituents of enzymes, hormones, and other compounds; are catalysts for reactions in the body; and are structural components of cells.

Calcium and iron are two minerals frequently deficient in the average American diet.

VITAMINS

Vitamins are essential for life but do not provide energy. They are necessary for release of energy from the energy nutrients. Individual vitamins are needed for specific metabolic reactions in the cell.

Vitamins are classified as the fat-soluble vitamins, including vitamins A, D, E, and K; and the water-soluble vitamins C and the B complex. Fat-soluble vitamins are stored in the body and do not need to be consumed daily since the body can use its stores. Water-soluble vitamins are not stored so some must be consumed daily. The B complex vitamins are a group of similar substances that are necessary for life. Thiamin, riboflavin, and niacin are the major B vitamins. Others include B_6 (pyridoxine), pantothenic acid, biotin, folacin, and B_{12} (cobalamin).

WATER

Approximately two-thirds of the body's weight is water. Water serves as a solvent and a transport medium for nutrients and waste products and is needed for reactions that occur in the body. Body fluids such as saliva, perspiration, blood, and digestive juices all contain water. Water is also a lubricant and helps regulate body temperature.

Water is supplied by fluids in the diet and many foods which contain a high percentage of water. Six to eight glasses of liquid daily are recommended. This amount varies, however, with factors such as climate and physical activity.

THE INDIVIDUAL MEAL PLAN

Because diet plays such a major role in the treatment of diabetes, it is important for the diabetic to follow his or her individual meal plan very carefully. This plan has been prescribed by a physician and/or a registered dietitian for the individual diabetic based on his weight, height, age, and level of activity. It shows what kinds of foods and the number of servings from each of the Exchange Lists that may be eaten at each meal in order to keep blood sugar within normal limits and to maintain a healthy body weight. By following the individual meal plan carefully, the diabetic will be certain to consume the correct number of calories, as well as the nutrients which are essential to maintaining good health.

EXCHANGE LISTS FOR MEAL PLANNING[1]

Since proper diet is the foundation for management of diabetes, it is important to plan each meal and snack with care. This can be done by learning the Exchange Lists and using them daily in accordance with the diabetic's meal plan. The Exchange Lists help control calories and carbohydrates while providing the variety of foods needed daily to supply all necessary nutrients. Weight-conscious members of your family can also use this method to count calories in groups of foods.

The Exchange List system for meal planning was developed many years ago by committees of the American Diabetes Association, the American Dietetic Association, and the United States Public Health Services. Changes have been made since the initial Lists were developed, and the Lists now include methods to reduce fat intake. Each List, or group of foods, contains similar amounts of protein, fat, carbohydrate, and calories. A food within each List can be traded or exchanged for any other food within that particular food group if eaten in the serving sizes listed.

[1]Exchange Lists for Meal Planning were prepared by the committees of the American Diabetes Association, Inc. and the American Dietetic Association in cooperation with the National Institute of Arthritis, Metabolism, and Digestive Diseases and the National Heart and Lung Institute, National Institutes of Health, Public Health Service, U.S. Department of Health, Education, and Welfare. Printed with permission.

The six Exchange Lists or food groups include:

1. Milk Exchanges   4. Bread Exchanges
2. Vegetable Exchanges   5. Meat Exchanges
3. Fruit Exchanges   6. Fat Exchanges

Recent research has shown that foods high in saturated fats tend to raise fat and cholesterol blood levels, a result which may increase the risk for heart disease. Foods high in polyunsaturated fats do not appear to raise fat and cholesterol blood levels; in fact, these fats sometimes tend to lower these levels. To serve as a guide, all foods which appear in **bold type** in the Exchange Lists are non-fat or low saturated-fat foods. Eating more of these foods in proportion to other foods is recommended not only for diabetics but for everyone.

MILK EXCHANGES
(Includes **Non-fat,** Low-fat, and Whole Milk)

One Exchange of Milk contains 12 grams of carbohydrate, 8 grams of protein, a trace of fat, and 80 calories.

This List shows the kinds and amounts of milk or milk products to use for one Milk Exchange. Those which appear in **bold type** are **non-fat.** Low-fat and Whole Milk contain saturated fat.

NON-FAT FORTIFIED MILK

Skim or non-fat milk	1 cup
Powdered (non-fat dry, before adding liquid)	⅓ cup
Canned, evaporated-skim milk	½ cup
Buttermilk made from skim milk	1 cup
Yogurt made from skim milk (plain, unflavored)	1 cup

LOW-FAT FORTIFIED MILK

1% fat fortified milk
  (omit ½ Fat Exchange)   1 cup
2% fat fortified milk
  (omit 1 Fat Exchange)   1 cup
Yogurt made from 2% fortified milk (plain, unflavored) (omit 1 Fat Exchange)   1 cup

WHOLE MILK (omit 2 Fat Exchanges)

Whole milk	1 cup
Canned, evaporated whole milk	½ cup
Buttermilk made from whole milk	1 cup
Yogurt made from whole milk (plain, unflavored)	1 cup

VEGETABLE EXCHANGES

One Exchange of Vegetables contains about 5 grams of carbohydrate, 2 grams of protein, and 25 calories.

This List shows the kinds of **vegetables** to use for one Vegetable Exchange. One Exchange is ½ cup.

Asparagus	**Greens**
Bean Sprouts	**Spinach**
Beets	**Turnip**
Broccoli	**Mushrooms**
Brussels Sprouts	**Okra**
Cabbage	**Onions**
Carrots	**Rhubarb**
Cauliflower	**Rutabaga**
Celery	**Sauerkraut**
Eggplant	**String Beans**
Green Pepper	**green or**
Greens	**yellow**
Beet	**Summer Squash**
Chards	**Tomatoes**
Collards	**Tomato Juice**
Dandelion	**Turnips**
Kale	**Vegetable Juice Cocktail**
Mustard	**Zucchini**

The following **raw vegetables** may be used as desired:

Chicory	**Lettuce**
Chinese Cabbage	**Parsley**
Endive	**Radishes**
Escarole	**Watercress**

Starchy Vegetables are found in the Bread Exchange List.

FRUIT EXCHANGES

One Exchange of Fruit contains 10 grams of carbohydrate and 40 calories.

This List shows the kinds and amounts of **fruits** to use for one Fruit Exchange.

Apple	1 small
Apple Juice	⅓ cup
Applesauce (unsweetened)	½ cup
Apricots, fresh	2 medium
Apricots, dried	4 halves
Banana	½ small
Berries	
Blackberries	½ cup
Blueberries	½ cup
Raspberries	½ cup
Strawberries	¾ cup
Cherries	10 large
Cider	⅓ cup
Dates	2
Figs, fresh	1
Figs, dried	1
Grapefruit	½
Grapefruit Juice	½ cup
Grapes	12
Grape Juice	¼ cup
Mango	½ small
Melon	
Cantaloupe	¼ small
Honeydew	⅛ medium
Watermelon	1 cup
Nectarine	1 small
Orange	1 small
Orange Juice	½ cup
Papaya	¾ cup
Peach	1 medium
Pear	1 small
Persimmon, native	1 medium

Pineapple	½ cup
Pineapple Juice	⅓ cup
Plums	2 medium
Prunes	2 medium
Prune Juice	¼ cup
Raisins	2 tablespoons
Tangerine	1 medium

Cranberries may be used as desired if no sugar is added.

BREAD EXCHANGES
(Includes **Bread**, **Cereal**, and **Starchy Vegetables**)

One Exchange of Bread contains 15 grams of carbohydrate, 2 grams of protein, and 70 calories.

This List shows the kinds and amounts of **Breads**, **Cereals**, **Starchy Vegetables** and Prepared Foods to use for one Bread Exchange. Those which appear in **bold type** are **low-fat**.

Bread

White (including French and Italian)	1 slice
Whole Wheat	1 slice
Rye or Pumpernickel	1 slice
Raisin	1 slice
Bagel, small	½
English Muffin, small	½
Plain Roll, bread	1
Frankfurter Roll	½
Hamburger Bun	½
Dried Bread Crumbs	3 tablespoons
Tortilla, 6″	1

Cereal

Bran Flakes	½ cup
Other ready-to-eat unsweetened Cereal	¾ cup
Puffed Cereal (unfrosted)	1 cup
Cereal (cooked)	½ cup
Grits (cooked)	½ cup
Rice or Barley (cooked)	½ cup
Pasta (cooked), Spaghetti, Noodles, Macaroni	½ cup

Popcorn (popped, no fat added)	3 cups
Cornmeal (dry)	2 tablespoons
Flour	2½ tablespoons
Wheat Germ	¼ cup

Crackers

Arrowroot	3
Graham, 2½-inch square	2
Matzoth, 4- x 6-inch	½
Oyster	20
Pretzels, 3⅛-inch long x ⅛-inch diameter	25
Rye Wafers, 2- x 3½-inch	3
Saltines	6
Soda, 2½-inch square	4

Dried Beans, Peas, and Lentils

Beans, Peas, Lentils (dried and cooked)	½ cup
Baked Beans, no pork (canned)	¼ cup

Starchy Vegetables

Corn	⅓ cup
Corn on Cob	1 small
Lima Beans	½ cup
Parsnips	⅔ cup
Peas, Green (canned or frozen)	½ cup
Potato, White	1 small
Potato (mashed)	½ cup
Pumpkin	¾ cup
Winter Squash, Acorn or Butternut	½ cup
Yam or Sweet Potato	¼ cup

Prepared Foods

Biscuit, 2-inch diameter (omit 1 Fat Exchange)	1
Corn Bread, 2- x 2- x 1-inch (omit 1 Fat Exchange)	1
Corn Muffin, 2-inch diameter (omit 1 Fat Exchange)	1
Crackers, round butter type (omit 1 Fat Exchange)	5
Muffin, plain small (omit 1 Fat Exchange)	1
Potatoes, French Fried (length 2-inch to 3½-inch) (omit 1 Fat Exchange)	8

Potato or Corn Chips (omit 2 Fat Exchanges)	15
Pancake, 5- x ½-inch (omit 1 Fat Exchange)	1
Waffle, 5- x ½-inch (omit 1 Fat Exchange)	1

MEAT EXCHANGES
Low-fat Meat

One Exchange of Lean Meat (1 ounce) contains 7 grams of protein, 3 grams of fat, and 55 calories. To plan a diet low in saturated fat and cholesterol, choose only those exchanges in **bold type**.

This List shows the kinds and amounts of **Lean Meat** and other protein-rich foods to use for one Low-fat Meat Exchange.

Beef:	**Baby Beef (very lean), Chipped Beef, Chuck, Flank Steak, Tenderloin, Plate Ribs, Plate Skirt Steak, Round (bottom, top), all cuts Rump, Sirloin, Tripe**	1 ounce
Lamb:	**Leg, Rib, Sirloin, Loin (roast and chops), Shank, Shoulder**	1 ounce
Pork:	**Leg (Whole Rump, Center Shank), Ham, Smoked (center slices)**	1 ounce
Veal:	**Leg, Loin, Rib, Shank, Shoulder, Cutlets**	1 ounce
Poultry:	**Meat without skin of Chicken, Turkey, Cornish Hen, Guinea Hen, Pheasant**	1 ounce
Fish:	**Any fresh or frozen**	1 ounce
	Canned Salmon, Tuna, Mackerel, Crab and Lobster	¼ cup
	Clams, Oysters, Scallops, Shrimp	5 or 1 ounce
	Sardines, drained	3
Cheeses containing less than 5% butterfat		1 ounce
Cottage Cheese, Dry and 2% butterfat		¼ cup
Dried Beans and Peas (omit 1 Bread Exchange)		½ cup

Medium-fat Meat

One Exchange of Medium-fat Meat (1 ounce) contains 7 grams of protein, 5 grams of fat, and 75 calories.

For each Exchange of Medium-fat Meat omit ½ Fat Exchange.

This List shows the kinds and amounts of Medium-fat Meat and other protein-rich foods to use for one Medium-fat Meat Exchange.

Beef:	Ground (15% fat), Corned Beef (canned), Rib Eye, Round (ground commercial)	1 ounce
Pork:	Loin (all cuts Tenderloin), Shoulder Arm (picnic), Shoulder Blade, Boston Butt, Canadian Bacon, Boiled Ham	1 ounce
Liver, Heart, Kidney, and Sweetbreads (these are high in cholesterol)		1 ounce
Cottage Cheese, creamed		¼ cup
Cheese:	Mozzarella, Ricotta, Farmer's cheese, Neufchatel	1 ounce
	Parmesan	3 tablespoons
Egg (high in cholesterol)		1
Peanut Butter (omit 2 additional Fat Exchanges)		2 tablespoons

High-fat Meat

One Exchange of High-fat Meat (1 ounce) contains 7 grams of protein, 8 grams of fat, and 100 calories.

For each Exchange of High-fat Meat omit 1 Fat Exchange.

This List shows the kinds and amounts of High-fat Meat and other protein-rich foods to use for one High-fat Meat Exchange.

Beef:	Brisket, Corned Beef (Brisket), Ground Beef (more than 20% fat), Hamburger (commercial), Chuck (ground commercial), Roasts (Rib), Steaks (Club and Rib)	1 ounce

Lamb:	Breast	1 ounce
Pork:	Spare Ribs, Loin (Back Ribs), Pork (ground), Country-style Ham, Deviled Ham	1 ounce
Veal:	Breast	1 ounce
Poultry:	Capon, Duck (domestic), Goose	1 ounce
Cheese:	Cheddar types	1 ounce
Cold Cuts:	4½- x ⅛-inch slice	1 slice
Frankfurter:		1 small

FAT EXCHANGES

One Exchange of Fat contains 5 grams of fat and 45 calories.
This List shows the kinds and amounts of Fat-containing Foods to use for one Fat Exchange. To plan a diet low in Saturated Fat select only those Exchanges which appear in **bold type**. They are **polyunsaturated**.

Margarine, soft, tub or stick*	1 teaspoon
Avocado (4" in diameter)**	⅛
Oil, Corn, Cottonseed, Safflower, Soy, Sunflower	1 teaspoon
Oil, Olive**	1 teaspoon
Oil, Peanut**	1 teaspoon
Olives**	5 small
Almonds**	10 whole
Pecans**	2 large whole
Peanuts**	
Spanish	20 whole
Virginia	10 whole
Walnuts	6 small
Nuts, other**	6 small
Margarine, regular stick	1 teaspoon
Butter	1 teaspoon

*Made with corn, cottonseed, safflower, soy, or sunflower oil only.
**Fat content is primarily monounsaturated.
***If made with corn, cottonseed, safflower, soy, or sunflower oil, dressing can be used on fat-modified diet.

Bacon fat	1 teaspoon
Bacon, crisp	1 strip
Cream, light	2 tablespoons
Cream, sour	2 tablespoons
Cream, heavy	1 tablespoon
Cream cheese	1 tablespoon
French dressing***	1 tablespoon
Italian dressing***	1 tablespoon
Lard	1 teaspoon
Mayonnaise***	1 teaspoon
Salad dressing, mayonnaise type***	2 teaspoons
Salt pork	¾-inch cube

*Made with corn, cottonseed, safflower, soy, or sunflower oil only.
**Fat content is primarily monounsaturated.
***If made with corn, cottonseed, safflower, soy, or sunflower oil, dressing can be used on fat-modified diet.

ADDITIONAL EXCHANGE LISTS[2]

SOUP EXCHANGES

Soups are made according to package directions using water or skim milk; when directions call for milk, the values include skim milk.

Beef (with vegetables and barley)	1 cup	½ Bread, ½ Meat
Cream of Chicken	1 cup	½ Bread, 1 Fat
Cream of Mushroom	1 cup	½ Bread, 2 Fats
Cream of Tomato	1 cup	1½ Bread
Chicken Gumbo	1¼ cups	½ Bread
Chicken Noodle, Beef Noodle	1 cup	½ Bread
Chicken with Rice	1¼ cups	½ Bread, ½ Meat
Clam Chowder, New England, made with skim milk	1 cup	1 Milk, ½ Bread

[2]Additional Exchange Lists from *A Guide to Meal Planning*. Printed with permission from the Birmingham District Dietetic Association, Birmingham, Alabama, 1980.

French Onion, Chef's		
Kettle	1¼ cups	1 Bread
Green Pea	1 cup	1½ Bread, ½ Meat
Minestrone	1¼ cups	1 Bread, ½ Meat
Split Pea with Ham and		
Bacon	1¼ cups	2 Bread, 1 Meat
Tomato	1 cup	1 Bread
Vegetable	1 cup	1 Bread
Vegetable Beef	1¼ cups	½ Bread, ½ Meat
Vegetarian Vegetable	1¼ cups	1 Bread

MISCELLANEOUS FOODS ALLOWED
(IN LIMITED AMOUNTS)
(2 choices per meal)

A-1 Sauce	2 teaspoons
Butter Buds, dry	4 tablespoons
Catsup, regular	1 tablespoon
Catsup, sugar-free	2 tablespoons
Chili sauce	1 tablespoon
Cocoa	1 tablespoon
Cranberries, unsweetened	½ cup
Lemon or lime juice	2 tablespoons
Pimiento, canned	2 medium
Horseradish	2 tablespoons
Imitation bacon bits	½ teaspoon
Non-dairy coffee creamer	1 teaspoon per meal
Non-dairy whipped topping	2 tablespoons
Postum	1 teaspoon per meal
Prepared mustard	2 tablespoons
Sugarless gum	4 sticks
Soy sauce	2 tablespoons
Tomato sauce	1 tablespoon
Tomato puree	1 tablespoon
Vinegar	¼ cup
Worcestershire sauce	1 tablespoon
Yeast, brewers	2 teaspoons

DIETETIC FOODS ALLOWED
(IN LIMITED AMOUNTS)

	(Daily Limit)
Dietetic gelatin	½ cup
Dietetic jam, jelly, syrup	1 tablespoon
Dietetic low-calorie	
salad dressing	Amount equal to 20 calories

FREE FOODS

Artificially Sweetened Beverages
Tea, coffee, lemonade, Kool-Aid, carbonated drinks

Baking Aids
Baking powder, baking soda, cream of tartar, yeast, pure flavoring extracts, calorie-free nonstick cooking spray

Foods
Bouillon, consommé, fat-free broth, dill or sour pickles, unflavored gelatin

Seasonings
Salt, pepper, meat tenderizers, herbs, spices

FOODS TO AVOID

Concentrated Sweets
Sugar, honey, syrup, molasses, desserts, frosting, candy, jelly, jams, preserves, marmalade, chewing gum (regular), cranberry sauce, condensed milk, sugar-coated cereals

Beverages
Presweetened drink mixes, carbonated drinks made with sugar, sweetened fruit juices, alcoholic beverages (unless approved by physician)

Dietetic Foods
Dietetic candy, dietetic cake, dietetic cookies, dietetic ice cream, sugarless mints

FOODS FOR SICK DAYS

There may be times when the diabetic finds eating difficult or impossible because of illness or dental work; during these times, loss of appetite or nausea and vomiting may be experienced. It is especially important at this time for the diabetic to follow his or her individual meal plan.

The following guidelines, Exchanges, and recipe suggestions should help in managing a meal plan in the event of illness:

1. Continue to eat and to take the prescribed insulin dose when sick.

2. Follow the meal plan as closely as possible, but eat only foods which can be tolerated well.

3. Use soft foods or liquids as an alternative if the usual foods are not tolerated.

4. Eat all the foods in the meal plan from the Bread, Milk, and Fruit Exchanges. Foods from the Meat, Vegetable, and Fat groups may be omitted until the illness is over.

5. Process regular foods in a blender or a food processor to aid chewing or swallowing problems. Foods should be measured into serving sizes before they are blended.

6. Consume extra liquids when there is vomiting or diarrhea to keep the body's fluid level from getting out of balance.

7. Eat popsicles or regular gelatin and drink sweetened drinks if nausea and vomiting are severe and there is difficulty in eating the foods on the meal plan. Sweetened products, however, should only be eaten or drunk in small amounts over a long period of time.

8. Prepare for an illness by keeping special foods and drinks handy for sick days.

When illness makes following a regular diet impossible, the Sick Day Exchanges listed here may be of some help. (Recipes for starred items are found in the recipe section of this book.)

MEAT - For 1 Exchange use:

Baby meats	½ of a 3½-ounce jar
Baked Custard*	⅔ cup (omit ½ skim milk)
Baked Lemon Pudding*	½ cup (omit 1 Fat)
Banana Cream Pudding*	½ cup (omit ½ Bread)
Cheese	1 ounce
Cottage cheese	¼ cup
Dietetic pudding	½ cup (omit 1 Bread)
Egg, soft-cooked or poached	1
Eggnog*	1 cup (omit 1 Skim Milk)
2% milk	1 cup (omit 1 Bread)
Pumpkin Custard*	1 cup (omit 1 Bread)
Yogurt, plain low-fat	1 cup (omit 1 Bread)

Hints:
Add baby meats to soups.
Put cheese in soups, mashed potatoes, or on toast.

BREAD - For 1 Exchange use:

Banana Cream Pudding*	1 cup (omit 2 Meats)
Bread	1 slice
Cocoa*	1 cup (omit 1 Meat)
Cooked cereal	½ cup
Corn flakes	¾ cup
Dietetic pudding	½ cup (omit 1 Meat)
Graham crackers	3 2½-inch squares
Mashed potatoes	½ cup
2% milk	1 cup (omit 1 Meat)
Noodles	⅓ cup
Pumpkin Custard*	1 cup (omit 1 Meat)
Rice	⅓ cup
Saltine crackers	6 2-inch squares
Soups (**undiluted**)	
Beef noodle	1 cup
Chicken noodle	1 cup
Chicken with rice	1¼ cups (omit 1 Meat)
Cream of chicken	1 cup (omit 2 Fat)

Cream of mushroom	1 cup (omit 4 Fat)
Cream of tomato	⅓ cup
Green pea	⅓ cup
Tomato	½ cup
Vegetable	½ cup
Vegetable beef	½ cup (omit 1 Meat)
Vegetarian vegetable	½ cup

Hints:

Add crackers, noodles, or rice to soups.

Let crackers or cereal soften in milk.

If vomiting is serious, the following regular sweetened foods and drinks should be used for 1 Bread Exchange:

Cola-type soft drink	5 ounces
Fruit-flavored soft drink	4 ounces
Ginger ale	6 ounces
Ice cream	½ cup (omit 2 Fat)
Popsicle	½ of a twin pop
Sherbet	¼ cup

VEGETABLES - For 1 Exchange use:

Tomato Aspic*	½ cup
Tomato juice	½ cup
Vegetable juice	½ cup

FRUIT - For 1 Exchange use:

Applesauce Parfait*	½ cup
Baby fruits	½ of 4½-ounce jar
Baked Lemon Pudding*	½ cup (omit 1 Meat)
Pineapple Sherbet*	⅓ cup (omit 1 Fat)
Unsweetened applesauce	½ cup
Unsweetened fruit juices	
Apple, pineapple	⅓ cup
Grape, cranberry,	
prune	¼ cup
Reduced-calorie	
cranberry	¾ cup
Orange, grapefruit	½ cup

Hints:
Add fruit or fruit juice to yogurt.
Add fruit juice to unflavored gelatin.

If the diabetic cannot eat any other foods, the following regular sweetened foods should be used for 1 Fruit Exchange:

Cola-type soft drink	3 ounces
Fruit-flavored soft drink	3 ounces
Ginger ale	4 ounces
Ice cream	⅓ cup

FAT

Hint:
To use Fat Exchanges, add 1 teaspoon of margarine to pureed vegetables, mashed potatoes, or crackers.

MILK - For 1 Exchange use:

Baked Custard*	1⅓ cup (omit 2 Meats)
Cocoa*	1 cup
Dietetic pudding	½ cup
Eggnog*	1 cup (omit 1 Meat)
Powdered skim milk	⅓ cup of powder
Skim milk	1 cup
Tapioca Pudding*	⅔ cup
Yogurt, plain low-fat	1 cup (omit 1 Fat)
Yogurt Shake*	1 cup

Hint:
Use milk or powdered milk instead of water when making soups.

If the diabetic cannot eat any other foods, the following regular sweetened foods should be exchanged for 1 Milk Exchange:

Cola-type soft drink	4 ounces
Fruit-flavored soft drink	3 ounces
Ginger ale	5 ounces
Gelatin	½ cup

EATING AWAY FROM HOME

DINING OUT

Eating away from home can be pleasant and easy if the diabetic has learned the Exchange system and individual meal plan. Or the individual meal plan may be taken along to make selecting foods from the menu simpler. The diabetic should not hesitate to ask how foods are prepared. Fried foods, gravies, sauces, casseroles, and salad dressings should be avoided in favor of simply prepared foods whenever possible.

Practice in measuring foods will enable the diabetic to recognize correct portions and serving sizes. If serving sizes are too large, one may leave them on the plate, share with someone, or ask for a "doggie" bag.

The following guide offers some ideas to help in selecting the proper foods when dining out.

Appetizers. Clear broth, bouillon, or consommé are "free." Celery stalks, green pepper rings, radishes, and dill pickles may be eaten in moderation. Fresh fruit, soups, and juices need to be counted in Exchanges. Cream soups and creamed foods are not recommended.

Meat, Poultry, and Fish. Select broiled, baked, roasted, or grilled meat, fish, or poultry. If they are not on the menu, the diabetic may request them. Ask that gravy and sauces be omitted. Avoid casseroles, stews, and fried items. If fried breaded items are the only ones available, the outer coating should be removed before eating since most excess fat and carbohydrate are in the coating mixture. Trim meats of excess fat before eating.

Eggs. Poached, boiled, or scrambled eggs may be ordered. Fried eggs or eggs with sauces such as Eggs Benedict should be avoided.

Salads. Tossed salad, sliced tomatoes, sliced cucumber, or a lettuce wedge are good choices. Request that the salad dressing be served on the side rather than on the salad so the amount used can be controlled. Lemon wedges or vinegar are also good substitutes for salad dressing. The diabetic should avoid extras for tossed salads such as croutons and bacon bits unless they are counted as Exchanges in the meal plan.

Breads. Plain bread, rolls, toast, muffins, crackers, or breadsticks without butter are acceptable. Breads with a high fat content such as biscuits, cornbread, and hush puppies need to be counted as Fat Exchanges as well as Bread Exchanges.

Vegetables. Select plain raw, stewed, steamed, or baked vegetables prepared without fat. Avoid fried vegetables or vegetables with cream or cheese sauces.

Potatoes and Substitutes. Baked, steamed, or boiled potatoes are good selections if they are served without fats. Margarine, butter, sour cream, and bacon bits should be counted as Fat Exchanges. Plain steamed or boiled rice, noodles, or macaroni are also acceptable choices; fried, creamed, and scalloped items are not.

Desserts. Fresh fruit or unsweetened fruit juice may be requested if it is not on the menu; other desserts will contain sugar.

FAST FOODS

When work or travel requires eating in fast-food restaurants, the choices will be limited. Most fast-food items contain several Meat, Fat, and Bread Exchanges. If it is necessary to select fast foods, refer to page 181 for a listing of numerous fast foods and their Exchange values.

"BROWN BAGGING"

Sometimes it is easier to take meals and snacks along when eating away from home. Foods to meet the meal plan for the day can then be planned in advance. By preparing foods at home, leftovers, when available, can be used for bag meals and snacks.

When a refrigerator is available at work or school, a wide variety of foods can be taken and stored until mealtime. When no refrigeration is available, avoid taking foods which spoil quickly such as meat and egg salads, yogurt, cottage cheese, and puddings or custards containing eggs or milk.

What was left from last night's meal? Sliced roast beef, veal, or chicken are good for sandwiches. Cold leftover portions from several recipes found in this book also make good lunches: Oven-Fried Chicken, Hamburger Pizza, Deviled Eggs, and Salmon Loaf.

Some leftovers can be reheated and packed in a wide-mouth thermos to retain heat. Chili, Beef Stew, Macaroni and Cheese, Savory Hash, Turkey Hash, Vegetable Soup, and many other recipes found in this book can be packed this way.

Tuna Salad, Chunky Egg Salad, Chicken Salad, and Ham Salad can serve as a filling for bread or crackers. They can also be wrapped with a lettuce leaf or served in a green pepper or tomato shell. These cold foods can be carried in a wide-mouth thermos and should be refrigerated until used. Try canned fruits or salads such as Cole Slaw, Picnic Potato Salad, Carrot-Raisin Salad, or Waldorf Salad. Desserts such as Pumpkin Custard, Baked Lemon Pudding, Berry Pudding, Banana Cream Pudding, and Tapioca Pudding can also be kept cold in a wide-mouth thermos.

For variety, include items such as Apple Muffins, Cheese Straws, Cornmeal Muffins, Oatmeal Cookies, or Cinnamon Cookies instead of bread or crackers. Spiced Hot Tea and Cocoa will remain hot in a beverage thermos, while Yogurt Shake and Pear Shake can be kept cold in a thermos for meals or snacks.

Fresh fruits and vegetables in season are simple to prepare. Try apples, celery with cheese, cucumber slices with meat salad or sliced meat filling, and sliced meat wrapped around dill pickles or celery. These foods can be kept fresh in plastic bags or foil wrap.

By using imagination and planning, bag meals can contain a variety of delicious foods and also meet the diabetic's meal plan requirements.

PURCHASING FOODS

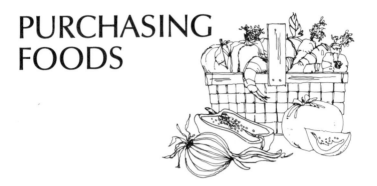

When there is a diabetic in the family, it becomes especially important to plan ahead and to buy proper yet economical foods. The diabetic's individual menu plan is based on sound principles of good nutrition which can be applied to all members of the family. A variety of foods from the various food groups provide the essential nutrients needed daily by all people throughout life. Adjustments can easily be made in food amounts consumed by each family member to meet each person's needs for body growth, maintenance, and energy. The following tips can help in selecting proper foods from each Food Exchange group.

SELECTION TIPS

MEAT EXCHANGES

- Buy plain meats, not ones frozen or canned in sauces.
- Buy frozen meats or fish that are not breaded.
- Buy meats and meat substitutes that are low in fat if you are trying to lose weight. Meat Exchanges high in fat include frankfurters, sausage, peanut butter, cheese, deviled ham, pork spare ribs, and beef brisket. Meat Exchanges low in fat include fresh fish, water-packed tuna, low-fat cheese, skinless chicken, turkey, round steak, flank steak, and lean ground beef.

BREAD EXCHANGES

- Buy plain cereals, not sugar-coated or granola-type cereals.
- Buy plain breads, not sweet breads such as coffee cake with icing.

- Buy breads and crackers low in fat if you or members of your family are trying to lose weight. High-fat breads include biscuits, cornbread, pancakes, waffles, taco shells, and snack crackers.

FRUIT EXCHANGES

- Buy fruit packed in its own juice or water, not fruits packed in heavy or light syrup. The fruit will absorb some of the sugar, and all of it cannot be rinsed off.
- Buy fresh fruits in season for best texture, flavor, and economy.
- Buy unsweetened fruit juices, not fruit-ade drinks or fruit punches. They contain mostly sugar, water, flavoring, and very little fruit juice.
- Buy frozen fruits which are unsweetened.

FAT EXCHANGES

- Buy reduced-calorie mayonnaise, reduced-calorie margarine, and reduced-calorie salad dressing if the diabetic or a family member is trying to lose weight. Generally, these have half the fat and calories of regular products.

MILK EXCHANGES

- Buy plain yogurt. Flavored yogurt usually contains sugars.
- Buy skim milk since it contains less fat than whole milk or low-fat milk.
- Do not buy sweetened condensed milk.
- Do not buy ice cream or ice milk. Although they are milk products, they contain too much sugar.

VEGETABLE EXCHANGES

- Do not buy vegetables packed in sauces.
- Do not buy frozen breaded vegetables.

DIETETIC FOODS

- Do not buy dietetic or "sugarless" foods. Dietetic products such as ice cream, cakes, and cookies contain flour and milk which are sources of carbohydrate and will affect blood glucose levels. Thus, even when a product is sugar-free, it usually cannot be used in unlimited amounts.

NUTRITION LABELING

Nutrition labeling acknowledges the consumer's right to know about the nutrient content of food and exactly what ingredients the consumer is purchasing. This information is helpful to all of us, but is especially valuable to diabetics. It is important to learn nutrients found in a food product and be able to convert the major nutrients into Exchanges if desired. For example, if a serving of a food product contains 2 grams of protein, 5 grams of fat and 15 grams of carbohydrate, one serving is equal to 1 Starch and 1 Fat Exchange. This type of information is useful when foods are not included in the Exchange Lists.

The following information is presently required on food labels: 1) nutrition information per serving (serving size, servings per container, amount of protein, carbohydrate, and fat); 2) percent of U.S. recommended daily allowances of protein, vitamin A, vitamin C, thiamin, riboflavin, niacin, calcium, and iron; and 3) a list of ingredients. The diabetic should notice two of these items in particular: serving size and ingredients. The food manufacturer determines the serving size listed on the label. This may need to be adjusted to fit the standard Exchanges. The listing of ingredients is very important to read for information and economy reasons. Sometimes water, sugar, or another ingredient which does not correspond to the name of the product is the major ingredient. For example, fruit drinks are primarily water, yet can be expensive. The first ingredient is always the main ingredient; the remaining ingredients are listed in order of their quantity in the product. Recommended Daily Allowances (RDA's) for selected nutrients are listed as the percentage of RDA that is provided by each serving of that food.

In addition to the food labeling required by law, the consumer may also run into terms like "dietetic," "calorie-controlled," or "sugar restricted" on food labels. These products may still contain some form of sugar. Dietetic products which contain milk and flour may also affect blood glucose levels because they are sources of carbohydrate. Avoid these products unless they do not contain any form of sugar.

If food labels are confusing, ask a registered dietitian to translate the values of protein, fat, and carbohydrate into Exchanges. Most companies provide nutrient analysis of their products upon request, but these values must be translated into Exchanges before they may be used in the diabetic's meal plan.

SUGAR

While sugar is not recommended for diabetics and weight-conscious individuals, its presence is often difficult to detect. Although most people equate "sugar" with household white or brown table sugar, many other forms exist. All sugars provide carbohydrate which affects blood glucose levels and should be avoided. In addition, many so-called "sugarless" products contain sweeteners such as sorbitol, xylotol, or mannitol which can affect blood glucose levels. Thus, even when a product is sugar free, it usually cannot be used in unlimited amounts. There are a number of terms which may appear on food labels to indicate that a product contains sugar. In order to avoid sugar in any form, it is important for the diabetic to know the words meaning sugar. The following is a list of words commonly found on labels that indicate sugar is an ingredient.

Brown Sugar: a soft sugar in which the crystals are covered by a film of refined dark syrup.

Carbohydrate: a term for sugars and starches.

Corn Sugar: sugar made by the breakdown of cornstarch.

Corn Syrup: a syrup containing several different sugars that is obtained by the partial breakdown of cornstarch.

Dextrin: a sugar formed by the partial breakdown of starch.

Dextrose: another name for sugar.

Fructose: the sweet sugar found in fruit, juices, and honey.

Glucose: a type of simple sugar found in the blood, derived from food, and used by the body for heat and energy.

Honey: a sweet, thick material made in the honey sac of various bees.

Invert Sugar: a combination of sugars found in fruits.

Lactose: the sugar found in milk.

Levulose: another name for fruit sugar.

Maltose: a crystalline sugar formed by the breakdown of starch.

Mannitol: a sugar alcohol.

Maple Sugar: a syrup made by concentrating the sap of the sugar maple.

Molasses: the thick syrup that is separated from raw sugar in sugar manufacture.

Sorbitol: a sugar alcohol.

Sorghum: syrup from the juice of the sorghum grain grown mainly for its sweet juice.

Starch: a powdery complex chain of sugars; for example, cornstarch.

Sucrose: another name for table sugar.

Sugar: a carbohydrate, including the monosaccharides: fructose, galactose, and glucose—and the disaccharides: sucrose, maltose, and lactose.

Xylotol: a sugar alcohol.

SUGAR SUBSTITUTES

Since table sugar (sucrose), the most commonly used sweetening agent, is not recommended for diabetics and weight-conscious individuals, many sugar substitutes have been developed. The recipes in this cookbook were designed to use these sugar substitutes.

These substitutes do not have the same properties as sucrose but do help to give foods a sweet taste. They do not provide the desired properties for browning, lightness, and tenderness in some foods. Often, sugar substitutes undergo chemical changes when heated, causing a bitter taste in the finished product. Each individual should try various brands and amounts to find a sugar substitute which provides the desired sweetness with minimum bitterness and aftertaste to meet the family's needs.

Refer to page 179 for a listing of several brands and recommended substitution equivalents for sugar.

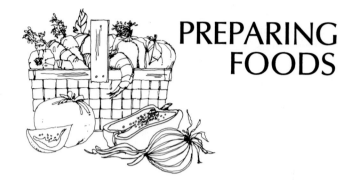

PREPARING FOODS

Foods must be cooked properly to enable the diabetic to follow the individual meal plan. Cooking with ingredients such as herbs or spices can make meals appetizing and food preparation a pleasure. The flavor and appearance of foods can be improved without adding extra calories. The following guidelines will assist in preparing food that is appropriate for the diabetic in the family.

PREPARATION HINTS

MEATS
- Bake, broil, roast, boil, or stew meats without adding fat. Do not fry.
- Trim meats of excess fat before cooking.
- Remove skin from poultry before cooking.

STARCHES
- Do not add fat when cooking rice or pasta, even when package directions advise adding fat.
- Count any fat added to cooked cereals, breads, or vegetables as Fat Exchanges.

VEGETABLES
- Boil, bake, or steam vegetables. Do not fry.
- Do not put creams or sauces over vegetables unless they are included in the individual meal plan.

- Cook vegetables without added fat such as oil, butter, margarine, bacon, bacon grease, fatback, cream, etc.; use the allowed Fat Exchanges to season vegetables at the table.
- Season vegetables with bouillon, lemon juice, herbs and spices, or butter substitute flavorings.

FRUITS

- Do not add sugars or syrups to fruits.
- To add flavor to water-packed fruit, try the following method: Drain fruit but reserve liquid, add 1 or 2 teaspoons lemon juice and sugar substitute, as desired, to the reserved liquid, pour liquid back over fruit, cover and store in refrigerator for 24 hours.

MILK

- Count any milk used in cooking as a Milk Exchange.

FATS

- Count all fat used in recipes as Fat Exchanges.

WEIGHING AND MEASURING HINTS

Follow these guidelines for measuring foods properly:
- Measure foods as they would be eaten with any bone, skin, fat, or inedible parts removed.
- Weigh meats on a scale designed for weighing foods.
- Measure vegetables, fruits, and cereals in dry measuring cups; fruits may also be weighed.
- Measure fluids in liquid measuring cups.
- Measure foods such as margarine, mayonnaise, peanut butter, and sour cream in teaspooons and tablespoons.

NOTE: When measuring food in cups or spoons, be sure the food is level with the top and not heaping. Measuring food will help the diabetic to eat the right amounts of protein, fat, carbohydrate, and calories. A registered dietitian can suggest the correct measurements to use for different foods, or you can refer to an Exchange List for diabetic diets.

NONSTICK COOKWARE

It is recommended that you use nonstick cooking ware for the recipes in this cookbook. When using nonstick cooking utensils, fats and oils do not need to be used for "greased" or "oiled" skillets, pans, and casserole dishes. Regular cooking ware can be converted to a nonstick surface by spraying the ware with a vegetable coating spray available in markets.

USING HERBS AND SPICES

Flavor, aroma, and variety can be added to recipes by seasoning foods with herbs and spices instead of fats. With more than 100 seasonings to pick from, a simple meal can be changed into a tasty treat. Add seasonings to uncooked foods such as salad dressings, fruits, and salads a few hours before serving to blend flavors. Add them to cooked foods such as stews, soups, and crackers during the last hour of cooking for the best taste and aroma.

Spices come from the bark, root, fruit, and berry of plants. Common spices include cinnamon, ginger, and pepper. Herbs, such as bay leaves, dill, and parsley, come from the leaves of small shrubs. Usually ¼ teaspoon of dried herbs is added for every four servings of food.

Seasoning foods is an art which requires trying various herbs and spices in differing amounts so that the flavor of food is improved but not overpowered. The right herb or spice or combination for specific foods is the one that tastes right to you.

Seasoning shakers can be prepared by mixing a blend of several ground herbs and spices and placing these in a salt or spice shaker. The seasoning shaker may be used to flavor foods during cooking or prior to serving.

The following are two ideas for seasoning shakers.

Measure and mix together:	Measure and mix together:
2 teaspoons dry mustard	4 teaspoons onion powder
1 teaspoon thyme	2 teaspoons thyme
1 teaspoon sage	½ teapsoon dry mustard
½ teaspoon marjoram	½ teaspoon curry powder

For other suggestions for using herbs and spices, refer to page 187.

CANNING AND FREEZING WITHOUT SUGAR

Foods may be preserved by canning or freezing without sugar to add variety to meals all year long. Vegetables may be canned without sugar using directions in any cookbook. Fruits may also be canned without sugar but will differ somewhat from those canned with sugar, since sugar helps to hold the shape, texture, appearance, color, and flavor of the fruit. Try to avoid using sugar substitutes when canning fruits. Heating sugar substitutes produces chemical changes which tend to create a bitter taste. If you use sugar substitutes, add them just before serving.

To prevent browning when canning light-colored fruits, use ascorbic acid or citric acid mixtures which may be purchased at drug stores. Follow the manufacturer's directions or add ½ teaspoon crystalline ascorbic acid to each quart of fruit. Recipes may be adapted to make artificially sweetened fruit spreads. Jams made without sugar are thinner than products made with sugar. Pectin or gelatin may be used to prepare some of these items, since jams prepared without jelling agents require longer cooking. Make small amounts and store by refrigerating or freezing.

Fruits and vegetables can be successfully frozen to retain original color, flavor, and texture. Freezing temperature of 0 degrees or below will retard the growth of bacteria, molds, and yeasts and will also slow enzyme activity. Freezer compartments in refrigerators are below 32 degrees but seldom reach 0 degrees or below; it is recommended that foods be frozen in these compartments only for short periods of time. For long-term freezing of larger quantities of food, a home freezer is recommended.

Before freezing, choose first-quality, fresh foods. Fruits should be ready to eat when frozen. They should be packed dry without sugar, or you may add sugar substitute. To keep fruit from darkening, add ascorbic acid. Vegetables are frozen by blanching in boiling water, cooling with water, draining, and packing dry or with cold water. Only sweet or bell peppers do not need to be blanched before freezing. For successful freezing, choose the proper packaging. Freezer containers and paper should be moisture proof and vapor proof.

Use frozen foods within 6 to 12 months for best quality. Thaw most foods in freezer containers in the refrigerator or in a pan of cool water. Do not refreeze.

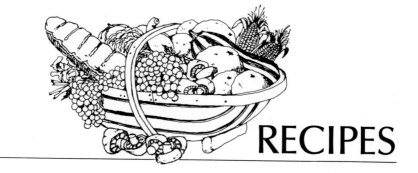

RECIPES

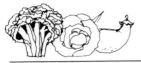

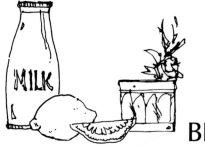

BEVERAGES

Beverages are an important part of regular meals but they may also be consumed between meals. Many beverages add little nutritive value to the diet. Some beverages contain sugar which should be omitted or replaced with a sugar substitute. Beverages do contain water which is a necesary nutrient for life, and at least eight glasses of water daily are recommended.

Coffee and tea usually contain a stimulant and may produce undesirable effects for some people. Beverages made with chocolate or cocoa add variety to meals.

Beverages with milk as the major ingredient add considerable nutrients to the diet, the greatest of which is the mineral calcium. To meet the body's needs for calcium, some milk or milk products should be included in the diet each day since calcium is found in only small amounts in other foods. The protein in milk is of high quality. Whole milk and fortified skim milk are excellent sources of Vitamins A and D. Milk is also very rich in the B vitamin riboflavin as well as some other B vitamins.

Some beverages may be made with fruit juice. The juice used determines the nutritive value and the proper Fruit Exchange. You may freeze some beverages to make slushes or "frozen pops" for variety.

Consider the nutritive and caloric value of a beverage when planning for a diabetic. The Exchange of a beverage should be worked into the meal plan.

FRESH LEMONADE OR LIMEADE

Yield: 2 servings	**Free Food**
Each Serving: 1 (8-ounce) glass	(Up to 4 glasses per day)

INGREDIENTS:

¼ cup fresh strained lemon
  or lime juice
Sugar substitute to equal 4
  teaspoons sugar
Cold water to make 2
  (8-ounce) cups

Fresh mint leaves and lemon
  or lime wedges
  (optional)

STEPS IN PREPARATION:
1. Combine juice and sugar substitute.
2. Add water, and stir well.
3. Add ice cubes as desired.
4. Garnish with mint leaves and lemon or lime wedges, if desired.

TROPICAL ICE

Yield: 24 servings	**One serving may be exchanged**
Each Serving: ½ cup	**for:** 1 Fruit

INGREDIENTS:

2½ cups unsweetened
  orange juice
2 cups mashed bananas
1 (20-ounce) can
  unsweetened crushed
  pineapple, undrained
1 tablespoon lemon juice

Sugar substitute to equal 1
  cup sugar
1 (32-ounce) bottle diet
  ginger ale
12 fresh strawberries
  (optional)

STEPS IN PREPARATION:
1. Combine orange juice, bananas, pineapple, lemon juice, and sugar substitute in large mixing bowl; stir well.
2. Freeze until firm.
3. To serve, let stand at room temperature until partially thawed.

4. Place in punch bowl, and break into chunks.
5. Add ginger ale, and stir until chunks soften.
6. Garnish with fresh strawberries, if desired, and serve.

HOLIDAY PUNCH

Yield: 6 servings	**One serving may be exchanged**
Each serving: 1 cup	**for:** ½ Fruit

INGREDIENTS:
    3½ cups diet lemon-lime   2 tablespoons lemon juice
      soda
    2½ cups reduced-calorie
      cranberry juice

STEPS IN PREPARATION:
1. Combine all ingredients in a large punch bowl.
2. Serve over ice.

TROPICAL FRUIT PUNCH

Yield: 11 servings	**One serving may be exchanged**
Each Serving: ½ cup	**for:** 1 Fruit

INGREDIENTS:
    3 cups unsweetened   2 teaspoons rum extract
      pineapple juice   Sugar substitute to equal ¼
    2 cups diet lemon-lime soda   cup sugar
    ½ cup unsweetened lime   Orange slices (optional)
      juice

STEPS IN PREPARATION:
1. Combine all ingredients except orange slices in large
   mixing bowl; mix well.
2. Serve over ice and garnish with orange slices, if desired.

CRAN-ORANGE PUNCH

Yield: 8 servings	One serving may be exchanged
Each Serving: ½ cup	for: 1 Fruit

INGREDIENTS:

1¼ cups reduced-calorie cranberry juice

1 (6-ounce) can unsweetened frozen orange juice concentrate, thawed and undiluted

Sugar substitute to equal ¼ cup sugar

2 cups diet lemon-lime soda

STEPS IN PREPARATION:

1. Combine cranberry juice, orange concentrate, and sugar substitute in a large bowl; stir well and chill.
2. Add soda to fruit juice mixture just before serving.
3. Serve over crushed ice.

YOGURT SHAKE

Yield: 4 servings	One serving may be exchanged
Each serving: ¾ cup	for: 1 Non-fat Milk

INGREDIENTS:

1½ cups fresh ripe or frozen strawberries, sliced

Sugar substitute to equal ¼ cup sugar

Dash of salt

2 teaspoons vanilla extract

½ teaspoon almond extract

2 (8-ounce) cartons plain low-fat yogurt

STEPS IN PREPARATION:

1. Place all ingredients except yogurt into medium-size bowl; mix well.
2. Chill at least 2 hours to blend flavors.
3. Place strawberry mixture and yogurt into blender, and blend on high until smooth.
4. Serve cold.

PEAR YOGURT SHAKE

Yield: 3 servings	**One serving may be exchanged**
Each serving: 1 cup	**for:** ½ Bread
	1 Fruit

INGREDIENTS:

1 (16-ounce) can
  unsweetened pears with
  liquid, chilled
1 (8-ounce) carton plain
  low-fat yogurt

1 teaspoon vanilla extract
Sugar substitute to equal ¼
  cup sugar
Dash of cinnamon
Ice cubes (optional)

STEPS IN PREPARATION:

1. Combine pears with liquid, yogurt, vanilla, sugar substitute, and cinnamon in blender or food processor; blend until smooth.
2. Serve immediately in chilled glasses.
3. Add ice cubes, if desired.

EGGNOG

Yield: 4 servings	**One serving may be exchanged**
Each serving: 1 cup	**for:** 1 Non-fat Milk
	1 Medium-fat Meat

INGREDIENTS:

4 eggs, well beaten
4 cups skim milk
1 teaspoon vanilla extract

Sugar substitute to equal ¼
  cup sugar
Nutmeg (optional)

STEPS IN PREPARATION:

1. Combine eggs, milk, vanilla, and sugar substitute in a large bowl; stir until smooth.
2. Sprinkle with nutmeg, if desired, and serve.

COCOA

Yield: 4 servings	One serving may be exchanged
Each serving: 1 cup	for: 1 Non-fat Milk

INGREDIENTS:

2 tablespoons cocoa	Sugar substitute to equal 8
¼ teaspoon salt	teaspoons sugar
1 cup water	1 teaspoon vanilla extract
3 cups skim milk	

STEPS IN PREPARATION:

1. Combine cocoa and salt in small saucepan.
2. Add water, and place over low heat or in top of double boiler.
3. Boil gently for 2 minutes, stirring constantly.
4. Add milk and sugar substitute.
5. Stir constantly until mixture comes to a boil; remove from heat immediately.
6. Add vanilla.
7. Stir and serve.

SPICED HOT TEA

Yield: 6 servings	Free Food
Each serving: ⅔ cup	

INGREDIENTS:

1 cinnamon stick	2 thin slices orange with
3 whole cloves	rind
Dash of nutmeg	4 cups water
2 thin slices lemon with rind	3 to 4 tea bags, as desired

STEPS IN PREPARATION:

1. Combine all ingredients except tea in heavy saucepan; simmer 10 minutes.
2. Add tea bags, and let steep to taste.
3. Remove tea bags, and serve hot.

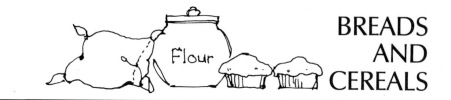

BREADS
AND
CEREALS

The major nutrient contribution of breads is carbohydrate for energy. When made from enriched flour, breads are also a source of iron and the B vitamins thiamin, riboflavin, and niacin. When milk is used in preparation, calcium and riboflavin are increased.

Flour used for baked products should be whole-grain flours when possible. During the milling and refining process, vitamins and minerals and the bran layer, which contains fiber, are removed. Although today's enriched flours contain added vitamins and minerals, fiber is not added. Because fiber may help control blood glucose, it is recommended that diabetics increase fiber in the diet. All members of the family need fiber for proper digestion and elimination.

Breads can be served to complement a meal. Quick breads, which contain baking powder or baking soda as the leavening agent, add interest to meals and include muffins, biscuits, cornbreads, and fruit breads. Dough for biscuits, a traditional favorite hot bread, should be handled just enough to knead or mix quickly; too much mixing makes biscuits tough. Cornbreads are also a favorite, especially in the South. The best cornbread is made from "water-ground" cornmeal which retains its germ layer and traditional flavor; however, it does not keep well. Processed cornmeal is highly refined and thus has better keeping qualities. Muffins, another favorite quick bread, can be varied by adding fruits, spices, and other ingredients to the basic mixture. Overmixing or beating makes tough, coarse-textured muffins. When using these breads, be sure to count as the correct Exchanges in the individual meal plan.

Most breads can be prepared in advance and stored in the freezer; they may be reheated as needed.

BISCUITS

Yield: 36 biscuits Each serving: 1 biscuit	Each serving may be exchanged for: 1 Bread 1 Fat

INGREDIENTS:

1 package dry yeast
2 tablespoons warm water
(105°-115°)
2 cups buttermilk
5 cups all-purpose flour

Sugar substitute to equal ¼
cup sugar
1 tablespoon baking powder
1 teaspoon soda
1 teaspoon salt
1 cup shortening

STEPS IN PREPARATION:

1. Combine yeast and warm water; let stand 5 minutes or until bubbly.
2. Add buttermilk to yeast mixture, and set aside.
3. Combine dry ingredients in large bowl; cut in shortening until mixture resembles coarse crumbs.
4. Add buttermilk mixture to dry mixture, stirring with fork until dry ingredients are moistened.
5. Turn dough out on floured surface, and knead lightly about 3 or 4 times.
6. Roll dough to ½-inch thickness; cut into 36 rounds with a 2-inch cutter, and place on nonstick baking sheets.
7. Bake at 400° for 10 to 12 minutes.

SPOONBREAD

Yield: 8 servings Each Serving: ½ cup	Each serving may be exchanged for: 1 Bread ½ Fat

INGREDIENTS:

1 cup plain cornmeal
1 teaspoon salt
1 cup water
2 cups hot skim milk

2 eggs, beaten
3 tablespoons
reduced-calorie
margarine, melted

STEPS IN PREPARATION:
1. Combine cornmeal and salt in medium saucepan.
2. Stir in water; gradually add hot milk, stirring until smooth.
3. Place over low heat, stirring constantly until thickened.
4. Spoon small amount of hot mixture into eggs; mix well.
5. Add egg mixture to remaining hot mixture, stirring constantly.
6. Add margarine; stir well.
7. Pour into nonstick 1½-quart baking dish.
8. Bake at 375° for 40 to 50 minutes.

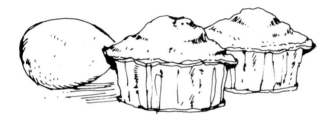

FRESH CORN MUFFINS

Yield: 8 muffins	**Each serving may be exchanged**
Each serving: 1 muffin	**for:** 2 Bread
	1 Fat

INGREDIENTS:

1 cup plain cornmeal
½ cup all-purpose flour
1 tablespoon plus 1
    teaspoon baking powder
1 teaspoon salt

1 cup fresh corn
1 egg, slightly beaten
¼ cup vegetable oil
1 cup buttermilk

STEPS IN PREPARATION:
1. Combine first 4 ingredients in medium mixing bowl.
2. Add corn, egg, oil, and buttermilk, stirring well.
3. Pour batter into 8 nonstick muffin cups.
4. Bake at 475° for 20 to 25 minutes or until brown.

PLAIN MUFFINS

Yield: 12 muffins
Each serving: 1 muffin

Each serving may be exchanged
for: 1 Bread
½ Fat

INGREDIENTS:

1½ cups sifted all-purpose
flour
3 teaspoons baking powder
½ teaspoon salt
1 egg, slightly beaten
½ cup skim milk

Liquid sugar substitute to
equal 2 tablespoons
sugar
4 tablespoons
reduced-calorie
margarine, melted

STEPS IN PREPARATION:

1. Sift flour, baking powder, and salt together into medium mixing bowl.
2. Add beaten egg, milk, and sugar substitute; add melted margarine when partially blended.
3. Pour batter into 12 nonstick muffin cups, filling each two-thirds full.
4. Bake at 400° for 20 to 25 minutes.

CORNMEAL MUFFINS

Yield: 12 muffins
Each serving: 1 muffin

Each serving may be exchanged
for: 1 Bread
½ Fat

INGREDIENTS:

1 cup plain yellow cornmeal
¾ cup sifted all-purpose
flour
½ teaspoon salt
1½ teaspoons baking
powder
½ teaspoon baking soda

Sugar substitute to equal 1
tablespoon sugar
1 medium egg, beaten
1 cup buttermilk
2 tablespoons
reduced-calorie
margarine, melted

STEPS IN PREPARATION:
1. Sift cornmeal, flour, salt, baking powder, baking soda, and sugar substitute together into medium mixing bowl.
2. Mix lightly with fork.
3. Combine beaten egg, buttermilk, and melted margarine; mix well.
4. Add egg mixture to cornmeal mixture.
5. Stir to mix well; then beat gently for 1 to 2 minutes.
6. Spoon 3 tablespoons batter into each of 12 nonstick muffin cups.
7. Bake at 400° for 25 to 30 minutes.

BRAN MUFFINS

Yield: 12 muffins **Each serving:** 1 muffin	**Each serving may be exchanged** **for:** 1 Bread ½ Fat

INGREDIENTS:

½ cup all-purpose flour
1 teaspoon baking soda
2 cups bran flakes
1 cup buttermilk
1 egg, slightly beaten

¼ cup reduced-calorie
   margarine, melted
Liquid sugar substitute to
   equal ¼ cup sugar
6 tablespoons raisins

STEPS IN PREPARATION:
1. Sift flour and soda together into medium-size mixing bowl; add bran flakes.
2. Combine buttermilk, egg, margarine, and sugar substitute.
3. Add milk mixture to dry ingredients, stirring only enough to mix ingredients slightly.
4. Add raisins.
5. Spoon 2½ tablespoons batter into each of 12 nonstick muffin cups.
6. Bake at 400° for 18 to 20 minutes.

APPLE MUFFINS

Yield: 12 muffins	**Each serving may be exchanged**
Each serving: 1 muffin	**for:** 1 Bread
	½ Fat

INGREDIENTS:

1⅔ cups all-purpose flour
2½ teaspoons baking powder
½ teaspoon salt
Sugar substitute to equal 1 tablespoon sugar
1 teaspoon cinnamon
¼ teaspoon nutmeg
1 egg, slightly beaten
⅔ cup skim milk
¼ cup reduced-calorie margarine, melted
1 cup apples, minced

STEPS IN PREPARATION:

1. Sift flour, baking powder, salt, sugar substitute, and spices into medium mixing bowl.
2. Combine egg, milk, and margarine.
3. Add egg mixture to dry ingredients, blending only until flour is moistened.
4. Fold in apples.
5. Pour batter into 12 nonstick muffin cups, filling each two-thirds full.
6. Bake at 400° for 25 minutes.

Always measure ingredients accurately. For liquids, use a glass measuring cup; this allows you to see that you are measuring correctly. Use metal or plastic dry measuring cups for solids; fill cups to overflowing, and level off with knife or metal spatula.

CRANBERRY-PECAN BREAD

Yield: 15 slices	**Each serving may be exchanged**
Each serving: 1 slice	**for:** 1½ Bread
	½ Fat

INGREDIENTS:

2 cups sifted all-purpose
    flour
1 teaspoon baking powder
1 teaspoon salt
½ teaspoon cinnamon
½ teaspoon nutmeg
1 egg
Liquid sugar substitute to
    equal 1 cup sugar
⅓ cup orange juice

1 teaspoon orange rind
3 tablespoons white vinegar
    plus enough water to
    make ⅔ cup
¼ cup reduced-calorie
    margarine, melted
1 cup coarsely chopped
    cranberries
24 small pecans, chopped

STEPS IN PREPARATION:

1. Sift together flour, baking powder, salt, cinnamon, and nutmeg into mixing bowl.
2. Beat egg; stir in sugar substitute, orange juice and orange rind, vinegar-water mixture, and margarine.
3. Add egg mixture all at once to flour mixture, and stir just until flour is moistened.
4. Add cranberries and pecans.
5. Spoon batter into nonstick 9- x 5- x 3-inch loafpan.
6. Bake at 350° for 60 to 70 minutes.
7. Cool in pan 10 minutes.
8. Remove from pan; cool overnight before slicing.
9. Slice into 15 equal slices.

Bread made with fruit or nuts should be tested with a straw or wire cake tester in the center. The tester should come out perfectly clean if the bread is done.

ORANGE MARMALADE NUT BREAD

Yield: 12 slices
Each serving: 1 slice

Each serving may be exchanged for: 1½ Bread
½ Fat

INGREDIENTS:

2 cups sifted all-purpose flour
1½ teaspoons baking powder
½ teaspoon baking soda
¼ teaspoon salt
½ cup skim milk
1 egg, slightly beaten
2 tablespoons reduced-calorie margarine, melted

Liquid sugar substitute to equal ½ cup sugar
1 teaspoon grated orange rind
½ cup dietetic orange marmalade
¼ cup chopped pecans

STEPS IN PREPARATION:

1. Combine flour, baking powder, soda, and salt in medium mixing bowl.
2. Combine milk, egg, margarine, sugar substitute, and orange rind in separate bowl.
3. Add milk mixture to flour mixture, stirring only until flour is moistened.
4. Fold in marmalade and nuts, stirring as little as possible.
5. Spoon batter into nonstick 9- x 5- x 3-inch loafpan.
6. Bake at 350° for 1 hour and 40 minutes.
7. Cool. Slice into 12 equal slices.

For ingredients listed in recipes: If the direction comes before the ingredient—for example, sifted flour—first sift the flour, then measure. If the direction comes after the ingredient—for example, pecans, chopped—first measure the pecans, then chop.

FRENCH TOAST

Yield: 2 servings	Each serving may be exchanged
Each serving: 2 slices	for: 2 Bread
	1 Medium-fat Meat

INGREDIENTS:

2 eggs   ¼ teaspoon salt

2 teaspoons skim milk   4 slices bread

STEPS IN PREPARATION:

1. Beat eggs.
2. Add milk and salt; beat until frothy.
3. Dip bread into egg mixture, thoroughly soaking each slice.
4. Place bread in nonstick skillet and brown slowly; turn and brown other side.

POTATO PANCAKES

Yield: 16 pancakes	Each serving may be exchanged
Each serving: 2 pancakes	for: 1 Bread
	½ Fat

INGREDIENTS:

3⅓ cups shredded cooked   2 tablespoons
   potatoes   reduced-calorie

2 eggs, beaten   margarine, melted

¾ cup skim milk   1 teaspoon salt

¼ cup chopped onion   1 teaspoon baking powder

2 tablespoons all-purpose
   flour

STEPS IN PREPARATION:

1. Combine potatoes and eggs; mix well.
2. Add remaining ingredients and blend well.
3. Let stand 10 minutes.
4. Drop batter, using ¼-cup measure, onto hot nonstick skillet; shape into circles.
5. Brown on one side; turn and brown on other side.

CORNBREAD DRESSING

Yield: 8 servings	**Each serving may be exchanged**
Each serving: ¾ cup	**for:** 1 Bread
	½ Fat

INGREDIENTS:

3 cups crumbled cornbread
1 cup bread crumbs
2 cups fat-free chicken broth
1 cup celery, finely chopped
¾ cup onion, finely
  chopped

2 egg whites
½ teaspoon salt
½ teaspoon pepper
½ teaspoon poultry
  seasoning

STEPS IN PREPARATION:

1. Combine all ingredients in mixing bowl; mix well.
2. Turn into nonstick baking dish.
3. Bake at 350° for 45 minutes or until light brown and "set".

CHEESE STRAWS

Yield: 48 straws	**Each serving may be exchanged**
Each serving: 3 straws	**for:** ½ Bread
	½ Fat

INGREDIENTS:

1 cup sifted all-purpose flour
½ teaspoon baking powder
½ cup reduced-calorie
  margarine
1 cup shredded low-fat
  process American cheese

3 tablespoons very cold
  water
⅛ teaspoon liquid pepper

STEPS IN PREPARATION:

1. Sift flour and baking powder into bowl.
2. Cut margarine and cheese into flour mixture until mixture resembles coarse meal.

3. Add water and pepper slowly to mixture.
4. Stir with a fork until all ingredients are moistened.
5. Chill mixture well for one hour in refrigerator.
6. Divide dough into 48 equal strips or fill cookie press and form 48 straws.
7. Place strips or straws on nonstick cookie sheets.
8. Bake at 375° for 8 to 10 minutes.
9. Place on wire racks to cool.

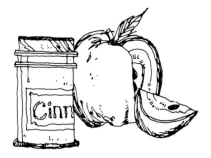

APPLE-CINNAMON OATMEAL

Yield: 3 servings
Each serving: ½ cup

Each serving may be exchanged for: 1 Bread
1 Fruit

INGREDIENTS:

1½ cups water
¼ teaspoon salt
⅔ cup quick-cooking oatmeal
1 medium apple, peeled and grated

1 teaspoon cinnamon
2 tablespoons raisins
Sugar substitute to taste

STEPS IN PREPARATION:

1. Bring water and salt to boil in saucepan.
2. Stir in oatmeal, apple, cinnamon, and raisins.
3. Reduce heat, and cook 1 minute until water is absorbed.
4. Serve hot with sugar substitute.

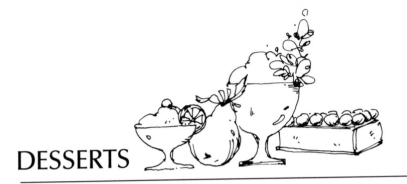

DESSERTS

Desserts are the sweet endings that complete a good meal. There are many varieties: Some light and low in calories, some containing many calories. Diabetics and others who must limit the amount of sugar they eat often do not have a wide variety of desserts available. However, with the proper substitution of ingredients such as sugar substitutes and reduced-calorie margarine in recipes, many favorite desserts can be included in the meal plan.

Desserts may be plain fresh fruits, cool puddings, or cakes. The nutrient content of the dessert depends on the ingredients used. Spices and flavoring extracts are important ingredients which can greatly enhance the flavor of the dessert. Try adding spices and flavorings to provide variety, and use reduced-calorie margarine and sugar substitutes in recipes. Reduced-calorie margarine can usually be substituted for butter or margarine in the same amounts. However, try different types and amounts of sugar substitutes to obtain the desired sweet taste and texture.

Choosing the right dessert is as much of an art as preparing it. Always choose a dessert that complements the menu. If a meal has been light, choose a baked dessert or a milk dessert such as pudding, custard, or cheesecake. If the meal has been heavy, select a light dessert such as fruit. Desserts chosen carefully can add important nutrients to the meal.

In this book are recipes for varied and traditional cookies, pies, puddings, and other desserts created especially for diabetics or weight-conscious members of the family. Be certain to count each serving in the correct Exchanges.

BAKED APPLES

Yield: 4 servings **Each serving:** 1 apple	**Each serving may be exchanged for:** 1 Fruit

INGREDIENTS:

4 small cooking apples
Sugar substitute to equal 8
   teaspoons sugar
½ teaspoon cinnamon

½ teaspoon nutmeg
1 cup water
1 tablespoon lemon juice, if
   desired

STEPS IN PREPARATION:

1. Wash and core apples; cut 1 small slice from the top and bottom of apples.
2. Place apples in small baking dish.
3. Combine remaining ingredients, and pour over apples.
4. Bake at 350° for about 45 minutes or until tender; baste every 15 minutes.

SPICED BAKED BANANAS

Yield: 6 servings **Each serving:** ½ banana	**Each serving may be exchanged for:** 1 Fruit

INGREDIENTS:

3 small, very ripe bananas,
   peeled
Brown sugar substitute to
   equal 4 teaspoons brown
   sugar

2 teaspoons grated lemon
   rind
⅛ teaspoon cinnamon
½ teaspoon vanilla extract

STEPS IN PREPARATION:

1. Place bananas in nonstick baking dish.
2. Sprinkle with brown sugar substitute, lemon rind, cinnamon, and vanilla.
3. Bake at 350° for 15 to 20 minutes.
4. Serve hot.

BAKED BANANAS ON THE HALF SHELL

Yield: 12 servings
Each serving: ½ banana

Each serving may be exchanged for: 1 Fruit

INGREDIENTS:

6 small bananas
¼ cup lemon juice
Brown sugar substitute to equal 6 tablespoons brown sugar

3 teaspoons reduced-calorie margarine
2 teaspoons rum extract

STEPS IN PREPARATION:

1. Slit unpeeled bananas in half lengthwise.
2. Place in baking dish, cut side up.
3. Sprinkle bananas with lemon juice and brown sugar substitute; dot with margarine.
4. Let stand several minutes.
5. Sprinkle with rum extract, and place under broiler 8 to 10 minutes; baste once or twice while broiling.
6. Serve hot.

GRAPEFRUIT SUPREME

Yield: 12 servings
Each serving: ¼ grapefruit

Each serving may be exchanged for: 1 Fruit

INGREDIENTS:

Sugar substitute to equal ½ cup sugar
¼ cup unsweetened orange juice

1 pint fresh strawberries, washed and hulled
3 large grapefruits cut in quarters

STEPS IN PREPARATION:

1. Combine sugar substitute and orange juice in medium-size bowl; mix well.
2. Stir in strawberries.

3. Refrigerate until thoroughly chilled.
4. Remove seeds from grapefruit quarters, and loosen sections.
5. Spoon strawberry mixture evenly over grapefruit, and serve.

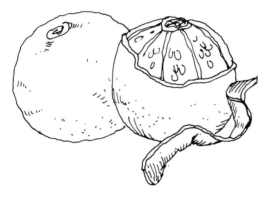

BRANDIED ORANGES

Yield: 12 servings **Each serving:** ¼ cup	**Each serving may be exchanged for:** 1 Fruit

INGREDIENTS:

3 large oranges
⅓ cup dark seedless raisins
¼ cup orange juice

1 teaspoon brandy extract
¼ cup slivered almonds, toasted

STEPS IN PREPARATION:

1. Peel oranges with sharp knife.
2. Section oranges and remove membrane.
3. Place in medium bowl.
4. Combine raisins, orange juice, and brandy extract.
5. Add brandy sauce to oranges.
6. Cover and refrigerate overnight to develop flavor; stir occasionally.
7. Sprinkle with almonds before serving.

CINNAMON ORANGES

Yield: 4 servings	Each serving may be exchanged
Each serving: ½ cup	for: 1 Fruit

INGREDIENTS:

Sugar substitute to equal ⅓ cup sugar

1½ teaspoons cinnamon

½ teaspoon cloves

4 medium oranges, peeled and thinly sliced

¼ cup water

½ teaspoon rum extract

STEPS IN PREPARATION:

1. Combine sugar substitute, cinnamon, and cloves in small bowl.
2. Arrange layer of overlapping orange slices in deep serving bowl.
3. Sprinkle with some of cinnamon mixture.
4. Continue layering oranges and cinnamon mixture.
5. Combine water and rum extract; pour over oranges.
6. Cover and refrigerate overnight.
7. Spoon juice over oranges to moisten before serving.

SPICED PEACH DESSERT

Yield: 3 servings	Each serving may be exchanged
Each serving: ½ cup	for: 1 Fruit

INGREDIENTS:

1 (16-ounce) can unsweetened peach halves

½ teaspoon cornstarch

⅛ teaspoon cinnamon

⅛ teaspoon cloves

Dash of nutmeg

½ teaspoon orange extract

Brown sugar substitute to equal 2 tablespoons brown sugar

STEPS IN PREPARATION:

1. Drain peaches, and reserve juice; set aside.

2. Combine cornstarch, cinnamon, cloves, and nutmeg in medium saucepan.
3. Stir in reserved peach juice until well blended.
4. Add peaches; bring to boil, stirring constantly.
5. Reduce heat, and simmer 2 minutes.
6. Remove from heat; add orange extract and brown sugar substitute, mixing well.
7. Serve warm.

BAKED GINGER PEARS

Yield: 8 servings **Each serving:** 2 halves	**Each serving may be exchanged** **for:** 1 Fruit 1 Fat

INGREDIENTS:

16 canned, unsweetened pear halves

Brown sugar substitute to equal 1 cup brown sugar

1 teaspoon ground ginger, divided

2 teaspoons lemon juice

½ cup chopped pecans

STEPS IN PREPARATION:

1. Drain pears and reserve juice; set aside.
2. Combine brown sugar substitute, ½ teaspoon ginger, lemon juice, and pecans.
3. Stuff pear halves with mixture; sprinkle with remaining ½ teaspoon ginger.
4. Place pear halves close together in nonstick baking dish.
5. Pour reserved pear juice into dish to cover bottom of dish.
6. Bake at 350° for 15 to 20 minutes.
7. Serve warm or chilled.

Organize your spice shelf and save much time by keeping the spices in alphabetical order. Store all spices in tightly covered containers to retain flavor and fragrance.

BAKED SPICED PEARS

Yield: 12 servings	Each serving may be exchanged
Each serving: ½ cup	for: 1 Fruit

INGREDIENTS:

6 medium fresh pears, peeled and sliced
Brown sugar substitute to equal ¾ cup brown sugar
2 tablespoons crystallized ginger
¼ teaspoon cinnamon
Dash of allspice
1½ teaspoons rum extract
2 teaspoons reduced-calorie margarine

STEPS IN PREPARATION:
1. Arrange pear slices in nonstick baking dish.
2. Combine brown sugar substitute, ginger, cinnamon, allspice, and rum extract.
3. Sprinkle brown sugar mixture over pears.
4. Dot pears with margarine.
5. Bake at 350° for 20 minutes.
6. Serve warm or chilled.

AMBROSIA

Yield: 5 servings	Each serving may be exchanged
Each serving: ½ cup	for: 1 Fruit

INGREDIENTS:

2 medium oranges, peeled
1 small banana, peeled
20 seedless green grapes, halved
¼ cup coconut

STEPS IN PREPARATION:
1. Cut oranges into small pieces.
2. Cut banana into very fine slices.
3. Combine all ingredients and serve.

FRESH FRUIT MEDLEY

Yield: 4 servings Each Serving: ½ cup	Each serving may be exchanged for: 1 Fruit

INGREDIENTS:

1 medium orange, peeled
½ medium grapefruit,
  peeled
1 small apple, cored
½ teaspoon fresh lime juice
  (optional)

Sugar substitute to equal 2
  teaspoons sugar
  (optional)
½ small banana, sliced

STEPS IN PREPARATION:

1. Section orange and grapefruit; cut into bite-size pieces.
2. Dice apple, and add to citrus fruit.
3. Sprinkle with lime juice and sugar substitute, if desired.
4. Chill for 1 hour or more.
5. Add banana to mixture just before serving.

FRUIT MELBA

Yield: 7 servings Each serving: ½ cup	Each serving may be exchanged for: 1 Fruit

INGREDIENTS:

½ cup reduced-calorie
  cranberry juice
1 teaspoon cornstarch
4 drops almond extract

1 cup fresh or frozen
  unsweetened raspberries
3 cups cantaloupe balls

STEPS IN PREPARATION:

1. Blend cranberry juice with cornstarch in a small saucepan.
2. Cook over medium heat, stirring constantly until mixture is
  thick and bubbly.
3. Remove sauce from heat; stir in almond extract, and cool.
4. Combine raspberries with cantaloupe balls; spoon ½ cup
  fruit into sherbet glasses.
5. Top with cooled sauce.

BANANA CREAM PUDDING

Yield: 4 servings	**Each serving may be exchanged**
Each serving: ½ cup	**for:** ½ Bread
	1 Medium-fat Meat

INGREDIENTS:

3 eggs, separated
½ cup skim milk
½ cup water
1 tablespoon unflavored
    gelatin

Sugar substitute to equal 2
    teaspoons sugar
1 teaspoon vanilla extract
1 medium-size banana,
    peeled and mashed

STEPS IN PREPARATION:
1. Beat egg yolks with milk and water in top of double boiler until blended; stir in gelatin.
2. Cook, stirring constantly, over hot, not boiling, water 7 minutes or until gelatin dissolves and mixture coats spoon.
3. Remove from heat.
4. Stir in sugar substitute and vanilla.
5. Chill 30 minutes or until mixture thickens.
6. Blend in mashed banana.
7. Beat egg whites until they form soft peaks; gradually fold into thickened gelatin mixture.
8. Chill several hours or until firm.

BERRY PUDDING

Yield: 6 servings	**Each serving may be exchanged**
Each serving: ½ cup	**for:** 1 Fruit

INGREDIENTS:

3 cups fresh or frozen
    unsweetened berries,
    divided
3 tablespoons cornstarch
⅛ teaspoon salt
⅛ teaspoon cinnamon

1 cup water
½ teaspoon vanilla or
    almond extract
Sugar substitute to equal 1
    cup sugar

STEPS IN PREPARATION:
1. Combine 1 cup of berries, cornstarch, salt, cinnamon, and water in saucepan.
2. Cook over medium heat, until mixture thickens, stirring constantly.
3. Add vanilla or almond extract, remaining 2 cups berries, and sugar substitute; mix well.
4. Cool and serve.

Note: May be served with Whipped Topping (page 174).

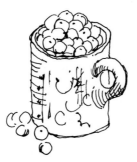

BLUEBERRY PUDDING

Yield: 4 servings	Each serving may be exchanged
Each serving: ½ cup	for: 1 Bread

INGREDIENTS:

1 cup crushed corn flakes	½ teaspoon vanilla extract
¼ teaspoon cinnamon	1 tablespoon melted
Sugar substitute to equal ¼	reduced-calorie
cup sugar	margarine
⅛ teaspoon salt	2 cups blueberries

STEPS IN PREPARATION:
1. Combine crushed flakes, cinnamon, sugar substitute, salt, vanilla, and melted margarine.
2. Place blueberries in bottom of baking dish; cover with corn flake mixture.
3. Bake at 350° for 20 minutes.

Note: May be served with Whipped Topping (page 174).

COCONUT BREAD PUDDING

Yield: 4 servings	**Each serving may be exchanged**
Each serving: ½ cup	**for:** 1 Bread
	1 Medium-fat Meat

INGREDIENTS:

2 cups skim milk

2 slices bread, crumbled

Sugar substitute to equal 3
  tablespoons sugar

2 eggs, slightly beaten

¼ cup coconut

½ teaspoon vanilla extract

STEPS IN PREPARATION:
1. Scald milk; add bread crumbs to milk.
2. Combine sugar substitute and eggs.
3. Add milk mixture slowly to egg mixture.
4. Stir in coconut and vanilla.
5. Pour into a nonstick casserole.
6. Place dish in pan of warm water.
7. Bake at 350° for 1 hour or until pudding is set.

BAKED LEMON PUDDING

Yield: 6 servings	**Each serving may be exchanged**
Each serving: ½ cup	**for:** 1 Non-fat Milk
	1 Fat

INGREDIENTS:

3 eggs, separated

Sugar substitute to equal ½
  cup sugar

¼ teaspoon salt

1½ cups skim milk

5 tablespoons all-purpose
  flour

⅓ cup plus 1 tablespoon
  lemon juice

¼ teaspoon lemon rind

2 tablespoons
  reduced-calorie
  margarine, melted

STEPS IN PREPARATION:
1. Combine egg whites, sugar substitute, and salt; beat until soft peaks form.
2. Combine egg yolks, milk, flour, lemon juice, lemon rind, and margarine; beat until smooth.
3. Fold in egg whites.
4. Pour into individual custard cups.
5. Place custard cups in pan of warm water.
6. Cover pudding loosely with aluminum foil.
7. Bake at 325° for 1 hour or until knife comes out clean when inserted in center.

TAPIOCA PUDDING

Yield: 6 servings	**Each serving may be exchanged**
Each serving: ⅓ cup	**for:** ½ Non-fat Milk

INGREDIENTS:

1 egg, separated	3 tablespoons tapioca
1¾ cups skim milk	½ teaspoon vanilla extract
Sugar substitute to equal 2	1 drop yellow food coloring
tablespoons sugar	

STEPS IN PREPARATION:
1. Combine egg yolk, milk, sugar substitute, and tapioca in medium saucepan.
2. Cook over low heat until mixture boils, stirring constantly.
3. Cool.
4. Add vanilla and food coloring.
5. Beat egg white until stiff; fold into tapioca mixture.
6. Spoon into serving dishes.

Always beat egg whites in a metal or glass container. Plastic retains fat and will interfere with foam formation.

BAKED CUSTARD

Yield: 2 servings **Each serving:** ⅔ cup	**Each serving may be exchanged** **for:** ½ Non-fat Milk 1 Medium-fat Meat

INGREDIENTS:

2 eggs	⅛ teaspoon salt
1 cup skim milk, scalded	½ teaspoon vanilla extract*
Sugar substitute to equal 2	Nutmeg (optional)
teaspoons sugar	

STEPS IN PREPARATION:

1. Beat eggs slightly.
2. Stir in scalded milk, sugar substitute, salt, and vanilla.
3. Pour into 2 custard baking cups; sprinkle with nutmeg, if desired.
4. Set cups in baking dish containing ½-inch hot water.
5. Bake at 325° for about 25 minutes or until silver knife inserted in center of custard comes out clean.
6. Serve warm or chilled.

*Note: For variety use lemon, orange, almond, or coconut flavoring in place of vanilla extract.

PUMPKIN CUSTARD

Yield: 6 servings **Each serving:** ½ cup	**Each serving may be exchanged** **for:** ½ Bread ½ Medium-fat Meat

INGREDIENTS:

2 eggs, well beaten	1½ teaspoons cinnamon
1½ cups skim milk	½ teaspoon allspice
1½ cups canned pumpkin	½ teaspoon ground cloves
Sugar substitute to equal 2	½ teaspoon ginger
tablespoons sugar	½ teaspoon nutmeg
⅛ teaspoon salt	

STEPS IN PREPARATION:
1. Mix all ingredients together, and blend well.
2. Pour into 6 custard baking cups.
3. Set cups in baking pan containing ½-inch hot water.
4. Bake at 425° for 10 to 15 minutes.
5. Reduce heat to 350° and bake for about 20 minutes or until knife inserted into center of custard comes out clean.
6. Serve either warm or chilled.

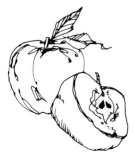

APPLESAUCE PARFAIT

Yield: 4 servings	**Each serving may be exchanged**
Each serving: ½ cup	**for:** 1 Fruit

INGREDIENTS:

1 envelope unflavored gelatin
2 tablespoons cold water
¼ cup boiling water
2 cups unsweetened applesauce

1 teaspoon cinnamon
⅛ teaspoon nutmeg
1 teaspoon vanilla extract
8 tablespoons Whipped Topping (page 174).

STEPS IN PREPARATION:
1. Place gelatin in small mixing bowl.
2. Add 2 tablespoons cold water, and let stand 5 minutes.
3. Add boiling water, and stir until gelatin is dissolved.
4. Add applesauce, cinnamon, nutmeg, and vanilla; mix well.
5. Layer ½ cup applesauce mixture with 2 tablespoons Whipped Topping in each of 4 parfait glasses.
6. Chill until served.

GRAPE FRAPPÉ

Yield: 4 servings	**Each serving may be exchanged**
Each serving: 1 cup	**for:** 1 Fruit

INGREDIENTS:

Sugar substitute to equal 1 cup sugar

2⅓ cups water

1 cup unsweetened grape juice

Juice of 2 fresh limes

STEPS IN PREPARATION:
1. Combine all ingredients in medium bowl; mix well.
2. Pour into freezer tray, and partially freeze.
3. Remove to chilled bowl.
4. Beat until fluffy and light in color.
5. Spoon into 4 serving cups and serve.

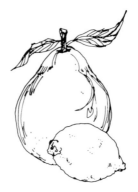

PEARSICLES

Yield: 4 servings	**Each serving may be exchanged**
Each serving: 1 pearsicle	**for:** 1 Fruit

INGREDIENTS:

1 (16-ounce) can unsweetened pears, undrained

3 tablespoons lime (or lemon) juice

½ teaspoon grated lime (or lemon) rind

4 paper cups

4 wooden stir sticks

STEPS IN PREPARATION:
1. Combine all ingredients in blender or food processor; blend until smooth.
2. Pour ½ cup mixture into each of 4 paper cups.
3. Freeze about 1 hour or until partially firm.
4. Insert wooden stick into each cup.
5. Freeze 2 to 4 hours or until firm.
6. Peel away cup before serving.

PINEAPPLE SHERBET

Yield: 4 servings	**Each serving may be exchanged**
Each serving: ½ cup	**for:** 1 Fruit
	1 Fat

INGREDIENTS:

Sugar substitute to equal 3
   tablespoons sugar
½ cup half-and-half
1⅓ cups unsweetened
   pineapple juice

4 egg whites
¼ teaspoon salt

STEPS IN PREPARATION:
1. Add sugar substitute to half-and-half, and freeze.
2. Freeze pineapple juice separately.
3. Combine frozen pineapple juice and frozen half-and-half mixture; beat until smooth.
4. Beat egg whites with salt until stiff but not dry.
5. Fold beaten egg whites into pineapple juice and half-and-half mixture.
6. Refreeze in 4 individual covered dishes until firm.

Raw eggs separate more easily while still cold from the refrigerator, but let whites reach room temperature to get maximum volume when beating.

VANILLA ICE CREAM

Yield: 6 servings	Each serving may be exchanged
Each serving: ½ cup	for: ½ Non-fat Milk
	2 Fat

INGREDIENTS:

1 tablespoon unflavored gelatin	Sugar substitute to equal ¼ cup sugar
1¼ cups skim milk, divided	2 teaspoons vanilla
2 eggs, separated	1 cup half-and-half
¼ teaspoon salt	

STEPS IN PREPARATION:

1. Soften gelatin in ¼ cup milk; set aside.
2. Combine remaining 1 cup milk, egg yolks, and salt in double boiler; heat until mixture coats spoon.
3. Remove from heat.
4. Add gelatin mixture and sugar substitute; stir until blended.
5. Cool.
6. Add vanilla and half-and-half.
7. Freeze until firm.
8. Beat egg whites until stiff peaks form.
9. Remove cream mixture from freezer, and place in chilled bowl; beat until smooth.
10. Fold in stiffly beaten egg whites.
11. Return to freezer until served.

To get maximum volume when beating cream, evaporated milk, or reconstituted dry milk, use a deep metal or glass bowl and have cream, bowl, and beaters very cold before starting.

DEEP-DISH APPLE PIE

Yield: 8 servings	**Each serving may be exchanged**
Each Serving: 1/8th of pie	**for:** 1½ Bread
	½ Fat

INGREDIENTS:

Sugar substitute to equal ⅓
   cup sugar
1 tablespoon cornstarch
½ teaspoon grated lemon
   rind
2½ teaspoons lemon juice
¼ teaspoon nutmeg
½ teaspoon cinnamon

4 small apples, sliced
1 cup all-purpose flour,
   sifted
1 teaspoon salt
¼ cup reduced-calorie
   margarine
3 tablespoons cold water

STEPS IN PREPARATION:

1. Combine sugar substitute, cornstarch, lemon rind, lemon juice, nutmeg, cinnamon, and apple slices.
2. Place in 9-inch deep-dish pie plate or baking dish; set aside.
3. Combine flour and salt; cut in margarine until mixture resembles cornmeal.
4. Blend in water with fork until all dry ingredients are moistened.
5. Shape dough into a ball.
6. Roll out dough on a floured surface, and place on top of apple filling.
7. Bake at 425° for 35 minutes or until brown.
8. Cut into 8 equal slices and serve.

Prices of fresh fruits and vegetables change with the seasons. Buy seasonal fresh foods when most plentiful and at peak quality in your area.

CHEESECAKE

Yield: 12 servings	Each serving may be exchanged
Each serving: 1 slice	for: 1 Non-fat Milk
	1 Fat

INGREDIENTS:

2 teaspoons unflavored gelatin

2 tablespoons cold water

Sugar substitute to equal ⅓ cup sugar

2½ cups low-fat cottage cheese

1 teaspoon vanilla

1 (16-ounce) can water-packed cherries

2 teaspoons cornstarch

Sugar substitute to equal ¼ cup sugar

⅛ teaspoon almond extract

6 drops red food coloring

14 graham cracker squares, crushed

4 tablespoons reduced-calorie margarine, melted

Sugar substitute to equal 1 tablespoon sugar

STEPS IN PREPARATION:

1. Combine gelatin and cold water in custard cup; let stand 1 minute.
2. Set cup in ½-inch boiling water to dissolve gelatin; remove from water and let cool.
3. Add sugar substitute equaling ⅓ cup sugar to cooled gelatin.
4. Combine cottage cheese and vanilla in blender, and blend until smooth.
5. Gradually add gelatin mixture to cottage cheese mixture.
6. Place mixture in bowl, and chill about 20 minutes or until slightly thickened; stir occasionally.
7. Meanwhile, drain cherries and reserve liquid.
8. Mix cornstarch and cherry liquid in small saucepan; stir until smooth.
9. Cook over medium heat, stirring constantly, until cherry mixture comes to a boil.
10. Reduce heat and cook 1 minute.
11. Remove from heat, and stir in cherries.

12. Cool to lukewarm, and blend in sugar substitute equaling ¼ cup sugar, almond extract, and food coloring; set aside.
13. Combine graham cracker crumbs, margarine, and sugar substitute equaling 1 tablespoon sugar.
14. Press mixture firmly into 9-inch pie pan.
15. Spoon cottage cheese mixture into crust; top with cherry glaze.
16. Chill overnight.
17. Cut into 12 equal slices.

APPLESAUCE CAKE

Yield: 15 servings	Each serving may be exchanged
Each serving: 1 slice	for: 1½ Bread
	½ Fat

INGREDIENTS:

6 tablespoons reduced-calorie margarine, softened	2 cups all-purpose flour, sifted
Liquid sugar substitute to equal 1 cup sugar	1 egg, beaten
1 teaspoon baking soda	1 teaspoon cinnamon
1 cup cold unsweetened applesauce	½ teaspoon nutmeg
	½ teaspoon cloves
	6 tablespoons raisins
	6 small walnuts, chopped

STEPS IN PREPARATION:

1. Cream margarine with sugar substitute.
2. Combine soda and applesauce, and add to margarine mixture.
3. Add remaining ingredients; stir just until blended. (Do not overmix.)
4. Pour into nonstick 7- x 11-inch baking pan.
5. Bake at 350° for 40 to 50 minutes.
6. When cake is cool, cut into 15 equal slices.

FRUIT CAKE

Yield: 16 individual cakes	**Each serving may be exchanged**
Each serving: 1 cake	**for:** 1½ Bread
	1½ Fat

INGREDIENTS:

½ cup orange juice, unsweetened

Liquid sugar substitute to equal 1½ cups sugar

1 cup fresh cranberries, finely chopped or 1 cup water-packed sour cherries, drained and finely chopped

1 cup seedless raisins

1 cup pecans, finely chopped

1 cup unsweetened pineapple chunks, drained and chopped

1 tablespoon grated orange rind

3 tablespoons reduced-calorie margarine, melted

1½ cups sifted all-purpose flour

1 teaspoon baking soda

½ teaspoon salt

¼ teaspoon allspice

¼ teaspoon cinnamon

¼ teaspoon nutmeg

STEPS IN PREPARATION:

1. Pour orange juice and sugar substitute over chopped cranberries.
2. Let stand for 1 hour.
3. Add raisins, pecans, pineapple, and orange rind to cranberry mixture.
4. Add melted margarine.
5. Sift and measure flour.
6. Add soda, salt, allspice, cinnamon, and nutmeg to flour; sift again.
7. Add dry ingredients to fruit mixture, and stir until thoroughly mixed.
8. Pour mixture into 16 nonstick baking cups.
9. Bake at 325° for 30 to 35 minutes until lightly browned.

APPLESAUCE COOKIES

Yield: 4 dozen	Each serving may be exchanged
Each serving: 3 cookies	for: 1 Bread
	½ Fat

INGREDIENTS:

1¾ cups cake flour
½ teaspoon salt
1 teaspoon cinnamon
½ teaspoon nutmeg
½ teaspoon ground cloves
1 teaspoon baking soda
½ cup reduced-calorie
 margarine

Liquid sugar substitute to
 equal ½ cup sugar
1 teaspoon vanilla extract
1 egg
1 cup unsweetened
 applesauce
⅓ cup raisins
1 cup bran cereal

STEPS IN PREPARATION:

1. Sift together flour, salt, cinnamon, nutmeg, cloves, and baking soda.
2. Combine margarine, sugar substitute, vanilla, and egg; cream until light and fluffy.
3. Add flour mixture and applesauce alternately to creamed mixture, mixing well after each addition.
4. Fold in raisins and bran cereal.
5. Drop 48 level tablespoons of cookie dough about 1 inch apart onto nonstick baking sheet.
6. Bake at 375° for 15 to 20 minutes or until golden brown.

Check foods closely as you are shopping to be sure they are not spoiled before you purchase them. Do not buy cans that are badly dented, leaking, or bulging at the ends. Do not select presealed packages which have broken seals.

CHOCOLATE-NUT BROWNIES

Yield: 16 brownies **Each serving:** 1 brownie	**Each serving may be exchanged** **for:** ½ Bread 1 Fat

INGREDIENTS:

⅓ cup plus 1 tablespoon
   reduced-calorie
   margarine, melted
Liquid sugar substitute to
   equal 1 cup sugar
3 teaspoons vanilla

2 eggs, beaten
2 tablespoons cocoa
1 cup sifted cake flour
½ teaspoon salt
½ teaspoon baking powder
12 pecans, finely chopped

STEPS IN PREPARATION:

1. Combine margarine, sugar substitute, vanilla, and eggs.
2. Sift together cocoa, flour, salt, and baking powder.
3. Add to liquid mixture; stir just until well blended. (Do not overmix.)
4. Stir in nuts.
5. Pour into nonstick 8-inch square pan; level batter in pan.
6. Bake at 325° for 20 minutes.
7. Cool on wire rack; cut into 16 squares.

CINNAMON COOKIES

Yield: 30 cookies **Each serving:** 3 cookies	**Each serving may be exchanged** **for:** ½ Bread ½ Fat

INGREDIENTS:

1 cup sifted all-purpose flour
¼ teaspoon baking powder
5 tablespoons
   reduced-calorie
   margarine

2 teaspoons vanilla extract
Liquid sugar substitute to
   equal ⅓ cup sugar
1 tablespoon orange juice
1 teaspoon cinnamon

STEPS IN PREPARATION:

1. Sift flour and baking powder together into mixing bowl.
2. Combine margarine and vanilla; cream until light and fluffy.
3. Blend flour mixture into creamed mixture.
4. Combine sugar substitute and orange juice.
5. Stir juice into flour mixture; mix dough well.
6. Sprinkle cinnamon over dough, and knead to make a streaked appearance.
7. Shape dough into 30 balls about one-half inch in diameter; arrange on nonstick cookie sheet.
8. Flatten balls with fork dipped in cold water.
9. Bake at 350° for 12 to 15 minutes or until edges are browned.

OATMEAL COOKIES

Yield: 24 cookies	**Each serving may be exchanged**
Each Serving: 1 cookie	**for:** 1 Bread

INGREDIENTS:

1½ cups all-purpose flour	½ teaspoon baking soda
1½ cups regular oatmeal, uncooked	¼ teaspoon salt
Sugar substitute to equal ½ cup sugar	¾ cup reduced-calorie margarine, softened
	3 tablespoons cold water

STEPS IN PREPARATION:

1. Combine all ingredients except margarine and water.
2. Cut margarine into dry mixture with pastry blender or knife; blend until mixture resembles coarse meal.
3. Sprinkle cold water evenly over surface; stir with fork until dry mixture is moistened.
4. Roll dough to ¼-inch thickness on waxed paper.
5. Cut into 24 rounds or squares.
6. Place cookies on nonstick cookie sheet.
7. Bake at 350° for 15 minutes.

SPICY OATMEAL COOKIES

Yield: 72 cookies **Each serving:** 2 cookies	**Each serving may be exchanged** **for:** ½ Bread ½ Fat

INGREDIENTS:

1½ cups quick-cooking
  oatmeal, uncooked
1 cup reduced-calorie
  margarine, melted
3 eggs, beaten
1 teaspoon vanilla extract
Liquid sugar substitute to
  equal 1¼ cups sugar
1¼ cups all-purpose flour,
  sifted

2 teaspoons baking powder
½ teaspoon salt
1 teaspoon cinnamon
1 teaspoon ground cloves
1 teaspoon nutmeg
½ cup skim milk
¼ cup raisins

STEPS IN PREPARATION:

1. Combine oatmeal and melted margarine in large mixing bowl; mix well.
2. Add eggs, vanilla, and sugar substitute to oatmeal mixture; stir until well blended.
3. Combine flour, baking powder, salt, cinnamon, cloves, and nutmeg in another bowl.
4. Add dry ingredients and milk alternately to oatmeal mixture; blend well.
5. Add raisins.
6. Set mixture aside 5 minutes.
7. Drop 72 level teaspoonsful onto nonstick cookie sheet.
8. Bake at 400° for 10 to 15 minutes or until golden brown.

Grills or pans with a nonstick finish may become scratched or lose their finish with use. Spray the damaged surface with a non-stick vegetable spray to prevent food from sticking.

LEMON-COCONUT COOKIES

Yield: 54 cookies	**Each serving may be exchanged**
Each serving: 4 cookies	**for:** 1 Bread
	1 Fat

INGREDIENTS:

½ cup reduced-calorie margarine

Liquid sugar substitute to equal ½ cup sugar

1 egg

1 tablespoon water

1 tablespoon grated lemon rind

1 tablespoon fresh lemon juice

1 teaspoon vanilla extract

½ cup shredded dry coconut

2 cups all-purpose flour, sifted

1 teaspoon baking powder

½ teaspoon salt

STEPS IN PREPARATION:

1. Cream margarine in small mixing bowl.
2. Add sugar substitute, egg, water, lemon rind, lemon juice, and vanilla; beat until well blended.
3. Add coconut, mixing well.
4. Sift flour, baking powder, and salt together.
5. Add to creamed mixture, mixing thoroughly on low speed if electric mixer is used.
6. Form dough into roll, 2 inches in diameter; wrap in waxed paper.
7. Chill until firm.
8. Cut into 54 thin slices, and place on nonstick cookie sheet.
9. Bake at 375° for 10 to 12 minutes or until lightly browned.

Get more juice from a lemon by heating it slightly in boiling water before squeezing.

EGGS
AND CHEESE

Eggs and cheese can be used together or separately to make many delicious foods. They are both good substitutes for meat in meals because the protein they contain is of excellent quality. Egg white is a rich source of the B vitamin riboflavin, while the yolk is a good source of iron and the vitamins A, E, B_6, B_{12}, and D. The nutrient value of eggs is not affected by the color of the shell, the size, or the grade. Most recipes require a medium egg unless otherwise specified. Grade AA or A are usually used for eating, while Grades B and C may be used in cooking and are less expensive.

In cooking with eggs, remember that the white cooks faster and at a lower temperature than the yolk. The white will be rubbery if cooked too long and at too high a temperature.

Cheeses contribute good quality protein and calcium to the diet and vary in nutritive value according to the kind of milk used, the moisture in the cheese, and the preparation of the cheese. Either whole or skim milk is used to make cheese. Whole-milk cheese has a higher fat content and thus provides more calories and vitamin A than cheeses made with skim milk. The moisture content of the cheese will affect the calorie content. The harder the cheese, the less moisture, and thus the more calories; whereas soft cheeses, such as cottage, have more moisture and fewer calories. There are many cheese foods or spreads available that contain added cream, non-fat dry milk solids, and other ingredients.

Domestic cheeses are usually less expensive than imported ones, although the nutritive value of cheese is not reflected by price. Sliced, shredded, or grated cheese will usually cost more than a wedge. Because the storage life of cheese is short once it has been cut or the package has been opened, plan to purchase only the amount which will be used in a short period of time.

EGG SALAD

Yield: 6 servings Each serving: ⅓ cup	Each serving may be exchanged for: 1 Medium-fat Meat

INGREDIENTS:

6 hard-cooked eggs, diced
½ cup diced celery
2 tablespoons minced green pepper
1 teaspoon minced onion
1 teaspoon salt
⅛ teaspoon pepper

2 tablespoons reduced-calorie mayonnaise
1 tablespoon vinegar
½ teaspoon Worcestershire sauce
Lettuce leaves (optional)

STEPS IN PREPARATION:

1. Combine all ingredients except lettuce; mix well.
2. Refrigerate until served.
3. Serve on lettuce leaf, if desired.

DEVILED EGGS

Yield: 4 servings Each serving: 2 egg halves	Each serving may be exchanged for: 1 Medium-fat Meat

INGREDIENTS:

4 hard-cooked eggs
½ teaspoon dry mustard
¼ teaspoon salt
Dash of onion powder
Dash of pepper

2 teaspoons reduced-calorie mayonnaise
1 teaspoon vinegar
Paprika

STEPS IN PREPARATION:

1. Halve eggs; remove yolks and mash.
2. Add other ingredients, except paprika, to mashed yolks; beat well.
3. Refill egg whites with yolk mixture.
4. Sprinkle with paprika.
5. Refrigerate until served.

EGGS BENEDICT

Yield: 4 servings	**Each serving may be exchanged**
Each serving: 1 muffin half	**for:** 1 Bread
	2 Medium-fat Meat

INGREDIENTS:

2 whole English muffins
4 (1-ounce) slices lean
   cooked ham
2 medium tomatoes, thickly
   sliced
4 eggs, poached and kept
   warm

6 tablespoons plain low-fat
   yogurt
1 teaspoon prepared
   mustard
Juice of ½ lemon

STEPS IN PREPARATION:

1. Slice muffins in half and toast.
2. On each half place 1 ham and 1 tomato slice.
3. Place under broiler 2 to 5 minutes.
4. Top each muffin half with poached egg.
5. Blend yogurt, mustard, and lemon juice.
6. Spoon 2 tablespoons sauce over each egg, and serve.

EGG-RICE CASSEROLE

Yield: 8 servings	**Each serving may be exchanged**
Each serving: 1/8th casserole	**for:** ½ Bread
	1 Medium-fat Meat

INGREDIENTS:

7 eggs, beaten
¾ cup skim milk
½ teaspoon celery salt
Dash of pepper

2 cups cooked rice
1 (4½-ounce) jar sliced
   mushrooms, drained

STEPS IN PREPARATION:
1. Combine first 4 ingredients; mix well.
2. Stir in rice and mushrooms.
3. Pour into nonstick 12- x 8- x 2-inch baking pan.
4. Bake at 350° for 30 to 35 minutes or until set.
5. Cut into 8 equal portions and serve.

DEVILED EGG CASSEROLE

Yield: 8 servings	**Each serving may be exchanged**
Each serving: 2 egg halves with	**for:** ½ Bread
¼ cup sauce	1½ Medium-fat Meat

INGREDIENTS:

8 hard-cooked eggs, cut in half

½ cup reduced-calorie mayonnaise

¼ cup chopped mushrooms

¼ teaspoon salt

2 tablespoons reduced-calorie margarine

2 tablespoons all-purpose flour

1½ cups skim milk

½ teaspoon Worcestershire sauce

1 cup shredded low-fat process American cheese

Paprika

STEPS IN PREPARATION:
1. Remove egg yolks and mash.
2. Combine yolks with mayonnaise, mushrooms, and salt.
3. Stuff egg whites with yolk mixture.
4. Place in nonstick 2-quart casserole, cut side up.
5. Melt margarine in nonstick skillet; stir flour in slowly.
6. Add milk and Worcestershire sauce very slowly, stirring constantly.
7. Add cheese, and stir until melted.
8. Pour mixture carefully over eggs.
9. Sprinkle with paprika.
10. Bake at 350° for about 30 minutes or until bubbly; serve.

HAM OMELET

Yield: 5 servings	**Each serving may be exchanged**
Each serving: 1/5th omelet	**for:** 2 Medium-fat Meat

INGREDIENTS:

8 eggs	1 tablespoon reduced-calorie
½ cup skim milk	margarine
1 teaspoon Italian seasoning	1 medium tomato, chopped
½ teaspoon salt	⅓ cup finely chopped
½ teaspoon pepper	cooked lean ham
6 drops liquid pepper	

STEPS IN PREPARATION:
1. Beat first 6 ingredients with fork until blended (do not overbeat).
2. Melt margarine in nonstick omelet pan; add blended egg mixture.
3. Begin cooking omelet on high heat; reduce to medium heat after a few minutes.
4. Add tomatoes and ham to top of one-half of omelet when eggs are partially set.
5. When eggs form light film on top, fold omelet in half and continue cooking until done.
6. Divide into 5 equal portions and serve.

BAKED EGGS AND MUSHROOMS

Yield: 4 servings	**Each serving may be exchanged**
Each Serving: 1/4th portion	**for:** 1 Medium-fat Meat
	1 Vegetable

INGREDIENTS:

4 eggs, beaten	1 cup cooked rice
½ cup skim milk	¼ cup sliced, canned
⅛ teaspoon salt	mushrooms, drained
Dash of pepper	

STEPS IN PREPARATION:
1. Combine eggs, milk, salt, and pepper; mix well.
2. Stir in rice and mushrooms.
3. Pour into 4 individual nonstick casseroles or an 8- x 8- x 2-inch nonstick baking dish.
4. Bake at 350° for 30 to 35 minutes.
5. If baked in baking dish, cut into 4 equal portions before serving.
6. Serve with Cheese Sauce, page 167.

EGGS IN CHEESE SAUCE

Yield: 8 servings **Each serving:** ⅓ cup	**Each serving may be exchanged** **for:** ½ Starch 1 Medium-fat Meat

INGREDIENTS:

1 (10¾-ounce) can cream of tomato soup
1½ cups shredded low-fat process American cheese
½ cup skim milk
½ cup sliced mushrooms, drained
1½ teaspoons reduced-calorie margarine
½ teaspoon Worcestershire sauce
⅛ teaspoon pepper
4 hard-cooked eggs, sliced

STEPS IN PREPARATION:
1. Place all ingredients, except eggs, in nonstick saucepan.
2. Bring to a boil while stirring constantly.
3. Gently stir in eggs, and serve.

Note: May be served over toast, rice, or noodles (count as a Bread Exchange).

Peel eggs from the large end, so shell will come off quickly.

CHEESE STRATA

Yield: 6 servings **Each serving:** 1/6th casserole	**Each serving may be exchanged** **for:** 1½ Bread 2 Low-fat Meat

INGREDIENTS:

6 slices bread, cubed 8 ounces low-fat process American cheese, shredded	3 eggs, beaten 2 cups skim milk ¼ teaspoon salt

STEPS IN PREPARATION:

1. Layer half of bread cubes in nonstick 1-quart casserole.
2. Layer half of shredded cheese on bread cubes; repeat layers.
3. Combine eggs, milk, and salt; pour over bread and cheese mixture.
4. Refrigerate several hours.
5. Set casserole in baking pan containing ½-inch of hot water.
6. Bake at 325° for 40 to 60 minutes or until knife inserted in center comes out clean.
7. Cut into 6 equal portions and serve.

BAKED CHEESE GRITS

Yield: 10 servings **Each serving:** ¼ cup	**Each serving may be exchanged** **for:** 1 Bread 1 Low-fat Meat

INGREDIENTS:

1 cup uncooked grits ⅓ cup skim milk 3 eggs, slightly beaten 8 ounces low-fat process American cheese, grated	½ teaspoon liquid pepper Salt to taste

STEPS IN PREPARATION:
1. Cook grits as directed on package.
2. Add, one ingredient at a time, milk, egg, cheese, pepper, and salt, mixing well after each addition.
3. Place in nonstick 1-quart casserole.
4. Bake at 325° until firm and slightly brown on top; serve immediately.

CHEESE SOUFFLÉ

Yield: 6 servings	**Each serving may be exchanged**
Each serving: ⅓ cup	**for:** 1 Bread
	1 Medium-fat Meat

INGREDIENTS:

4 slices bread, cubed	½ teaspoon salt
¾ cup skim milk	Dash of cayenne
1 cup grated low-fat process American cheese	½ teaspoon Worcestershire sauce
2 tablespoons reduced-calorie margarine	3 eggs, separated

STEPS IN PREPARATION:
1. Combine bread and milk in a heavy saucepan; bring mixture to a boil.
2. Add cheese, margarine, salt, cayenne, and Worcestershire sauce.
3. Beat egg yolks, and add slowly to mixture.
4. Beat well over medium heat; remove from heat.
5. Beat egg whites, and fold into mixture.
6. Place mixture in nonstick 1-quart casserole; place casserole in pan of water.
7. Bake at 400° for 35 to 40 minutes or until browned on top; serve immediately.

CHEESE-EGGPLANT SOUFFLÉ

Yield: 8 servings **Each serving:** ½ cup	**Each serving may be exchanged** **for:** 1 Medium-fat Meat 1 Vegetable

INGREDIENTS:

3 cups diced eggplant
½ teaspoon salt
3 eggs, slightly beaten
1 cup grated low-fat process
   American cheese

1 cup skim milk
1 tablespoon reduced-calorie
   margarine
⅛ teaspoon liquid pepper
Dash of pepper

STEPS IN PREPARATION:

1. Place eggplant in saucepan with water to cover.
2. Add salt, and cook until tender.
3. Drain and cool.
4. Combine with remaining ingredients.
5. Place mixture in nonstick 2-quart casserole.
6. Bake at 350° for 30 minutes; serve immediately.

SPINACH-CHEESE CASSEROLE

Yield: 5 servings **Each serving:** ½ cup	**Each serving may be exchanged** **for:** 1 Low-fat Meat 1 Vegetable

INGREDIENTS:

1 (10-ounce) package frozen
   chopped spinach
1 medium onion, chopped
2 teaspoons reduced-calorie
   margarine
1 cup low-fat cottage cheese

4 tablespoons grated low-fat
   process American
   cheese, divided
⅛ teaspoon nutmeg
Dash of pepper

STEPS IN PREPARATION:

1. Cook spinach according to directions on package; drain
spinach well.

2. In nonstick skillet, sauté onion in margarine until tender.
3. Add spinach, cottage cheese, 2 tablespoons grated low-fat cheese, nutmeg, and pepper; stir well.
4. Pour into nonstick 1-quart casserole.
5. Sprinkle with remaining grated cheese.
6. Bake at 350° for 25 to 30 minutes until set.

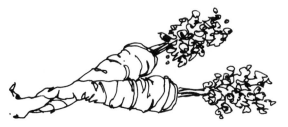

COTTAGE CHEESE-VEGETABLE CASSEROLE

Yield: 12 servings
Each serving: ½ cup

Each serving may be exchanged for: 1 Bread
1 Low-fat Meat

INGREDIENTS:

1 cup thinly sliced carrots
½ cup chopped onion
1 tablespoon reduced-calorie margarine
½ cup sliced mushrooms
1 (8-ounce) package noodles, cooked and drained

2 cups low-fat cottage cheese
½ cup skim milk
½ teaspoon salt
½ teaspoon basil
¼ teaspoon thyme
⅛ teaspoon pepper
Parsley sprigs (optional)

STEPS IN PREPARATION:

1. Combine carrots, onion, and margarine in non-stick skillet; cook on medium heat until tender.
2. Add mushrooms and cook 5 minutes; set aside.
3. Combine remaining ingredients, except parsley, in large bowl; stir in cooked vegetables.
4. Turn mixture into nonstick 2-quart casserole.
5. Cover and bake at 350° for 30 minutes or until bubbly.
6. Garnish with parsley before serving, if desired.

MACARONI AND CHEESE

Yield: 6 servings	**Each serving may be exchanged**
Each serving: ½ cup	**for:** 1 Bread
	1 Medium-fat Meat

INGREDIENTS:

1½ cups skim milk

1½ tablespoons all-purpose flour

1½ tablespoons reduced-calorie margarine

½ teaspoon salt

¾ cup grated low-fat process American cheese

2 cups macaroni, cooked and drained

¼ cup breadcrumbs

STEPS IN PREPARATION:

1. Combine milk, flour, margarine, and salt to make a white sauce (see page 167 for steps).
2. Return sauce to low heat.
3. Add grated cheese, stirring constantly.
4. Cook until cheese has melted and sauce boils.
5. Remove from heat.
6. Alternate layers of macaroni and cheese sauce in nonstick baking dish; cover top with breadcrumbs.
7. Bake at 375° until mixture bubbles and crumbs brown.

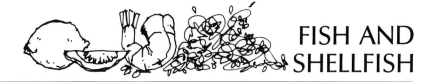

FISH AND SHELLFISH

Fish and shellfish are important sources of protein in the diet. Shellfish are especially high in the minerals iron and iodine, and they provide some B vitamins. Fish or shellfish may be used in appetizers and salads, as main dishes, and in casseroles.

Most fish and shellfish can be cooked by broiling, grilling, steaming, or baking. To avoid overcooking fish or shellfish, test for doneness by piercing with a fork. When the flesh flakes easily, the fish is done; if the fish is "elastic," more cooking is necessary.

When buying fresh fish, purchase from a reliable dealer shortly before preparation since fish is highly perishable. Always check the freshness of the fish when buying. The market forms of fish are: whole (as they come from the water); drawn (with only the entrails removed); dressed (scaled and eviscerated); steaks (crosscut sections of larger dressed fish); and fillets (sides of fish cut lengthwise away from the backbone).

Frozen fish should always be thawed in the refrigerator, not at room temperature. Place the frozen fish package in another paper or plastic wrap before placing in the refrigerator. The additional wrap keeps other foods from absorbing the odor of the fish as it thaws. Never refreeze fish once it has thawed, and cook fish within one to two days after it thaws.

BAKED FISH FILLETS

Yield: 12 servings	**Each serving may be exchanged**
Each serving: 1 ounce	**for:** 1 Low-fat Meat

INGREDIENTS:

1 (16-ounce) package frozen fish fillets (not breaded), thawed
2 tablespoons reduced-calorie margarine
1½ teaspoons lemon juice
½ teaspoon salt
¼ teaspoon paprika
Lemon slices (optional)

STEPS IN PREPARATION:
1. Place fillets, skin side down, in nonstick baking pan.
2. Dot with margarine; sprinkle with lemon juice, salt, and paprika.
3. Bake at 350° for 20 to 30 minutes or until fish flakes easily.
4. Serve with lemon slices, if desired.

BROILED FISH FILLETS

Yield: 9 servings	**Each serving may be exchanged**
Each serving: 1 ounce	**for:** 1 Low-fat Meat

INGREDIENTS:

¼ cup Italian reduced-calorie dressing
¼ teaspoon salt
Dash of pepper
½ teaspoon Worcestershire sauce
¾ pound fish fillets
1 lime, halved
2 green onions, chopped

STEPS IN PREPARATION:
1. Combine dressing, salt, pepper, and Worcestershire sauce; add fillets and marinate for two hours.
2. Drain fillets; place in broiling pan, and broil until flaky.

3. Squeeze juice of ½ lime over fillets; broil 1 minute.
4. Remove fillets from oven and sprinkle with juice from remaining ½ lime.
5. Sprinkle with green onions before serving.

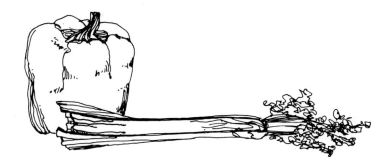

CREOLE FISH FILLETS

Yield: 8 servings **Each serving:** ½ cup	**Each serving may be exchanged** **for:** 1 Low-fat Meat 1 Vegetable

INGREDIENTS:

1 medium green pepper, chopped
¼ cup chopped onion
¾ cup sliced celery
1 tablespoon reduced-calorie margarine
1 (6-ounce) can tomato paste
1½ cups water
1 teaspoon salt
¼ teaspoon thyme
⅛ teaspoon pepper
1 bay leaf
Dash of garlic powder
2 cups diced, cooked fish fillets

STEPS IN PREPARATION:
1. Combine pepper, onion, and celery in nonstick skillet; sauté in margarine until tender.
2. Add tomato paste, water, and seasonings; simmer 15 minutes, stirring occasionally.
3. Add fish, and heat thoroughly.

Note: Serve over rice or noodles (count as a Bread Exchange).

ORIENTAL BROILED FISH

Yield: 12 servings **Each serving:** 1 ounce	**Each serving may be exchanged** **for:** 1 Medium-fat Meat

INGREDIENTS:

1 tablespoon salad oil
1 tablespoon soy sauce
1 clove garlic, crushed
⅛ teaspoon ground ginger

1 (16-ounce) package frozen
   fish fillets, thawed
2 tablespoons minced green
   onions

STEPS IN PREPARATION:

1. About 1½ hours before serving, combine oil, soy sauce, garlic, and ginger in bottom of broiling pan.
2. Place fillets in pan, and turn to coat with oil mixture.
3. Refrigerate 1 hour or more.
4. Broil 8 to 10 minutes or until fish flakes easily.
5. Sprinkle with green onions before serving.

OVEN-FRIED FISH

Yield: 6 servings **Each serving:** 2 ounces	**Each serving may be exchanged** **for:** ½ Bread 2 Low-fat Meat

INGREDIENTS:

½ cup crushed corn flakes
½ teaspoon celery salt
⅛ teaspoon onion powder
⅛ teaspoon paprika
Dash of pepper

1 pound catfish or other fish
   fillets
1 tablespoon plus 1
   teaspoon skim milk

STEPS IN PREPARATION:

1. Combine corn flakes, celery salt, onion powder, paprika, and pepper.
2. Dip fish in milk; roll in corn flake mixture.
3. Place fish in nonstick baking pan.
4. Bake at 350° for 25 minutes until brown.

FISH FILLET CASSEROLE

Yield: 9 servings	**Each serving may be exchanged**
Each serving: 3 ounces with	**for:** 2 Low-fat Meat
sauce	

INGREDIENTS:

1½ pounds fish fillets
1 (10¾-ounce) can cream of
    shrimp soup
¼ teaspoon liquid pepper

½ cup grated low-fat process
    American cheese
Paprika

STEPS IN PREPARATION:
1. Place fish in nonstick pan, skin side down.
2. Combine soup and liquid pepper; pour over fish.
3. Sprinkle with grated cheese and paprika; bake at 400° for 35 to 45 minutes.

SHRIMP SCAMPI

Yield: 10 servings	**Each serving may be exchanged**
Each serving: 2 ounces	**for:** 2 Low-fat Meat
	1 Vegetable

INGREDIENTS:

½ cup reconstituted dry
    butter substitute
½ teaspoon salt
½ teaspoon garlic powder
½ teaspoon parsley
¼ teaspoon oregano leaves
¼ teaspoon sweet basil

⅛ teaspoon cayenne pepper
1½ cups fat-free chicken
    broth
1½ tablespoons lemon juice
2 cups cooked shrimp,
    peeled and deveined
1 tablespoon cornstarch

STEPS IN PREPARATION:
1. Combine all ingredients except shrimp and cornstarch.
2. Bring to a boil and add shrimp.
3. Stir in cornstarch to thicken.

Note: Serve over rice or noodles (count as a Bread Exchange).

SHRIMP SALAD

Yield: 4 servings Each serving: ⅓ cup	Each serving may be exchanged for: 3 Low-fat Meat

INGREDIENTS:

1 pound fresh or frozen
  shrimp
⅛ teaspoon white pepper
¾ teaspoon chopped
  pimiento
⅛ teaspoon chopped parsley

¼ cup reduced-calorie
  mayonnaise
½ teaspoon prepared
  mustard
¾ teaspoon lemon juice
⅓ cup finely chopped celery

STEPS IN PREPARATION:

1. Place shrimp in boiling water to cover; cook 5 minutes.
2. Cool shrimp.
3. Peel and devein shrimp; chop.
4. Combine remaining ingredients except celery to make salad dressing; mix well.
5. Add shrimp and celery to salad dressing.
6. Refrigerate until served.

SEAFOOD NEWBURG

Yield: 6 servings Each serving: ¾ cup	Each serving may be exchanged for: 3 Low-fat Meat ½ Bread

INGREDIENTS:

1 pound frozen shrimp,
  peeled and deveined
¾ pound scallops
3 cups fat-free chicken broth
½ cup reconstituted dry
  butter substitute
½ teaspoon garlic powder
¼ teaspoon salt

¼ teaspoon white pepper
½ teaspoon parsley flakes
¼ teaspoon thyme
¼ teaspoon sage
3 tablespoons cornstarch
3 tablespoons water
2 tablespoons lemon juice

STEPS IN PREPARATION:
1. Cook shrimp and scallops in chicken broth 5 minutes.
2. Remove seafood and set aside.
3. Combine chicken broth, butter substitute, garlic powder, salt, white pepper, parsley flakes, thyme, and sage; heat to boiling.
4. Combine cornstarch and water; add to chicken broth mixture and simmer 5 minutes.
5. Add lemon juice; return shrimp and scallops to broth mixture, and serve.

TUNA CREOLE

Yield: 6 servings **Each serving:** 1 cup	**Each serving may be exchanged for:** 2 Low-fat Meat 1 Vegetable

INGREDIENTS:

1 cup chopped onions	1 (14½-ounce) can tomatoes
2 tablespoons chopped green pepper	¼ cup sliced stuffed olives
	½ teaspoon salt
2 tablespoons reduced-calorie margarine	½ teaspoon oregano
	⅛ teaspoon pepper
	⅛ teaspoon allspice
2 tablespoons all-purpose flour	2 (6½-ounce) cans water-packed tuna

STEPS IN PREPARATION:
1. Combine onions and green pepper in nonstick skillet; sauté in margarine until tender.
2. Add flour; mixing well.
3. Add tomatoes, olives, and seasonings; cook until thickened, stirring constantly.
4. Drain and flake tuna; stir into tomato mixture.

Note: Serve over rice or noodles (count as a Bread Exchange).

TUNA SALAD

Yield: 4 servings **Each serving:** ½ cup	**Each serving may be exchanged** **for:** 2 Low-fat Meat

INGREDIENTS:

1 (6½-ounce) can
  water-packed tuna
2 hard-cooked eggs,
  chopped
¼ cup chopped celery

2 tablespoons
  reduced-calorie
  mayonnaise
Lettuce leaves (optional)

STEPS IN PREPARATION:
1. Combine all ingredients except lettuce leaves.
2. Refrigerate until served.
3. Serve on lettuce leaf, if desired.

SALMON CROQUETTES

Yield: 5 servings **Each serving:** 1 croquette	**Each serving may be exchanged** **for:** 1 Bread 3 Low-fat Meat

INGREDIENTS:

1 (16-ounce) can salmon
⅔ cup skim milk
2 teaspoons reduced-calorie
  margarine
2 tablespoons minced onion
¼ cup all-purpose flour
¼ teaspoon salt

Dash of pepper
¾ teaspoon liquid pepper
1 tablespoon lemon juice
1 cup crushed corn flakes,
  divided
5 lemon wedges

STEPS IN PREPARATION:
1. Drain salmon, reserving liquid; add milk to reserved liquid.
2. Melt margarine in nonstick skillet; add onions and sauté until tender but not brown.
3. Add flour, salt, pepper, and liquid pepper to onion mixture; blend well.

4. Add milk mixture, and cook over low heat, stirring constantly, until thickened.
5. Flake salmon; add salmon and lemon juice to sauce.
6. Stir in ½ cup corn flakes.
7. Refrigerate until chilled.
8. Divide mixture into ½ cup portions, and shape into cones; roll cones in remaining corn flakes to coat well.
9. Place on nonstick baking sheet, and bake at 400° for 20 to 25 minutes or until golden brown.
10. Serve with lemon wedges.

SALMON LOAF

Yield: 4 servings	**Each serving may be exchanged**
Each serving: ½ cup	**for:** ½ Bread
	2 Low-fat Meat

INGREDIENTS:

½ cup skim milk
1½ slices bread, crumbled
1 cup canned salmon, flaked and drained
2 teaspoons lemon juice

¼ teaspoon salt
⅛ teaspoon paprika
⅛ teaspoon pepper
2 egg whites

STEPS IN PREPARATION:
1. Combine milk and bread; warm in top of double boiler or over very low heat.
2. Add flaked salmon, lemon juice, salt, paprika, and pepper.
3. Beat egg whites until stiff peaks form; fold into salmon mixture.
4. Place mixture in nonstick casserole.
5. Place casserole in pan of hot water.
6. Bake at 300° for 1 hour, and serve.

Note: Canned water-packed tuna may be substituted for salmon.

MEATS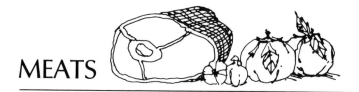

Frequently, meals are planned around the choice of meat, fish, or poultry, which are the greatest sources of protein in the diet. The protein content of meat depends on the source and cut of meat; as the amount of fat, bone, and connective tissue increases, the amount of protein decreases. The leaner the meat, the higher the protein content. To control calories, cholesterol, and saturated fats in the diet, choose lean meats and trim visible fat before cooking. Meat is an excellent source of iron as well as other minerals and some of the B vitamins.

Recipes in this section include beef, pork, veal, and specialty meats such as liver and frankfurters. Beef may be cooked by a variety of methods. Broiling and roasting are dry-heat methods which are used with tender cuts of meat such as sirloin and Porterhouse steak. Moist heat methods—braising and cooking in liquid—are used with less tender cuts of meat such as rump and chuck; moist heat softens tough connective tissues.

Most pork will be tender, so dry-heat cooking methods may be used. Pork should be cooked until completely done. Because veal is very low in fat content and contains much connective tissue, it should be cooked by moist heat for best results.

The flavor of meats may be altered by using various seasonings and herbs as suggested in the Spice and Herb Chart, pages 187-189. For economy, mix with other foods such as vegetables and starches in casseroles. Whenever using these mixed dishes, be sure to count the correct Exchanges in the meal plan.

MARINATED STEAK

Yield: 4 servings **Each serving:** 2 ounces steak with 2 tablespoons sauce	**Each serving may be exchanged for:** 2 Medium-fat Meat

INGREDIENTS:

1½ teaspoons
  Worcestershire sauce
4 (2½-ounce) round steaks
½ teaspoon garlic salt
½ teaspoon instant minced
  onion

½ teaspoon pepper
½ cup dry white wine
1 cup water
1 (3-ounce) can sliced
  mushrooms, drained

STEPS IN PREPARATION:

1. Spoon Worcestershire sauce over both sides of steaks.
2. Sprinkle steaks with next three ingredients.
3. Refrigerate 1 hour.
4. Place steaks in nonstick skillet; cook over medium heat, browning both sides.
5. Pour wine over steaks.
6. Cover and reduce heat to simmer; cook 15 minutes.
7. Remove steaks to serving platter and keep warm.
8. Add water and mushrooms to skillet; boil uncovered, stirring often, for about 10 minutes or until gravy is reduced to about ½ cup.
9. Pour gravy over steaks and serve.

When freezing meat patties, steaks, or chops, separate with two thicknesses of wrapping material between them so that the pieces can be separated without thawing more than needed.

STEAK DELUXE

Yield: 6 servings	**Each serving may be exchanged**
Each serving: 2 ounces steak	**for:** ½ Bread
with ¼ cup sauce	2 Medium-fat Meat

INGREDIENTS:

1 pound round steak, trimmed of fat	½ teaspoon vinegar
	½ teaspoon celery salt
2 tablespoons all-purpose flour	¼ teaspoon thyme
	⅛ teaspoon garlic powder
1 teaspoon reduced-calorie margarine	⅛ teaspoon pepper
	Brown sugar substitute to
1¼ cups cooked tomatoes	equal 1 tablespoon
½ medium onion, sliced	brown sugar
2 teaspoons Worcestershire sauce	

STEPS IN PREPARATION:
1. Pound flour into sides of steak.
2. Melt margarine in nonstick skillet.
3. Brown steak on both sides; remove steak to nonstick casserole.
4. Combine remaining ingredients; pour over steak.
5. Cover; bake at 300° for 2½ hours.
6. Uncover last 15 minutes to cook liquid to a thick sauce.
7. Serve hot with sauce.

SLICED STEAK AU JUS

Yield: 21 servings	**Each serving may be exchanged**
Each serving: 1 ounce	**for:** 1 Medium-fat Meat

INGREDIENTS:

1¾ pounds top round steak, trimmed of fat	Dash of pepper
	1 garlic clove, minced
1 (3-ounce) can sliced mushrooms, drained	1 tablespoon Worcestershire sauce
½ teaspoon salt	1 tablespoon lemon juice

STEPS IN PREPARATION:
1. Cut steak into ¼-inch slices; arrange slices in nonstick baking dish.
2. Sprinkle remaining ingredients over steak.
3. Cover with foil.
4. Bake at 350° for 1 hour; remove foil.
5. If necessary, bake 15 minutes longer or until steak is tender; baste occasionally.

BEEF STEW

Yield: 6 servings	**Each serving may be exchanged**
Each serving: 1 cup	**for:** 1 Bread
	2 Medium-fat Meat
	1 Vegetable

INGREDIENTS:

1 pound lean beef, cubed	2 cups boiling water
2 tablespoons	1 cup canned tomatoes
Worcestershire sauce	4 medium potatoes, cubed
½ teaspoon salt	3 medium carrots, sliced
¼ teaspoon oregano	3 small onions, quartered
⅛ teaspoon allspice	1 (10-ounce) package frozen
1 beef bouillon cube	peas

STEPS IN PREPARATION:
1. Marinate beef in Worcestershire sauce for several hours.
2. Brown beef cubes in nonstick skillet.
3. Add salt, oregano, and allspice.
4. Dissolve bouillon cube in boiling water; pour over beef.
5. Add tomatoes, and simmer over low heat 1½ to 2 hours or until meat is tender.
6. Add potatoes, carrots, and onions; continue to cook for 30 minutes.
7. Add peas; cook 15 minutes longer or until meat and vegetables are tender.

CHILI

Yield: 16 servings	Each serving may be exchanged
Each serving: ½ cup	for: ½ Bread
	1 Medium-fat Meat

INGREDIENTS:

½ cup chopped onion	1 (20-ounce) can kidney
1 pound lean ground beef	beans
1 teaspoon salt	3 cups water
1 tablespoon chili powder	
1 (20-ounce) can tomatoes	

STEPS IN PREPARATION:

1. Combine onion, ground beef, salt, and chili powder in nonstick skillet.
2. Cook on low heat until browned.
3. Combine tomatoes and beans in saucepan.
4. Add 3 cups water to make approximately 8 cups.
5. Add meat mixture.
6. Simmer slowly for 1 hour before serving.

GROUND BEEF PIE

Yield: 5 servings	Each serving may be exchanged
Each serving: 1½ cups with	for: 2 Bread
potatoes	2 Medium-fat Meat

INGREDIENTS:

1 pound lean ground beef	1 cup tomato juice
1 small onion, finely	1 (20-ounce) can green
chopped	beans*
1 teaspoon salt	2½ cups mashed potatoes
½ teaspoon chili powder	Paprika
⅛ teaspoon pepper	

STEPS IN PREPARATION:
1. Brown beef in nonstick skillet with onions, salt, chili powder, and pepper.
2. Drain fat.
3. Place mixture in nonstick 2-quart casserole.
4. Pour tomato juice over mixture.
5. Drain and place green beans on top of beef mixture.
6. Place 5 (½-cup) servings of mashed potatoes on top of green beans.
7. Sprinkle with paprika.
8. Bake at 350° for 35 to 40 minutes, and serve.

*Note: 3¾ cups fresh green beans may be used in place of canned green beans.

GROUND BEEF PIZZA

Yield: 6 servings	**Each serving may be exchanged**
Each serving: 1 wedge	**for:** 2 Medium-fat Meat

INGREDIENTS:

1 pound lean ground beef
1 teaspoon salt
¼ teaspoon pepper
1 cup canned tomatoes, well drained
2 tablespoons chopped parsley

2 tablespoons finely chopped onion
½ cup shredded low-fat process American cheese
2½ teaspoons Italian seasoning
¼ teaspoon allspice

STEPS IN PREPARATION:
1. Combine ground beef, salt, and pepper.
2. Pat meat into 9-inch nonstick pie pan.
3. Spread tomatoes over meat.
4. Combine remaining ingredients; sprinkle over tomato-meat mixture.
5. Bake at 350° for 20 minutes.
6. Cut into 6 equal wedges to serve.

SAVORY HASH

Yield: 6 servings	Each serving may be exchanged
Each serving: ½ cup	for: 2 Medium-fat Meat
	1 Vegetable

INGREDIENTS:

1 pound lean ground beef	1 teaspoon chili powder
½ cup finely chopped celery	¼ teaspoon pepper
½ cup finely chopped onion	2 cups tomatoes, fresh or
¼ cup finely chopped green	canned
pepper	½ cup cooked rice
1 teaspoon salt	

STEPS IN PREPARATION:

1. Combine ground beef, celery, onion, and green pepper in nonstick skillet; cook until meat is browned.
2. Drain accumulated fat.
3. Add salt, chili powder, pepper, tomatoes, and rice.
4. Cover and simmer over low heat for 45 minutes, adding water occasionally to keep meat from sticking to skillet.

ITALIAN SPAGHETTI

Yield: 4 servings	Each serving may be exchanged
Each serving: ½ cup sauce with	for: 1 Bread
½ cup spaghetti	1 Medium-fat Meat
	1 Vegetable

INGREDIENTS:

½ small onion, chopped	¼ teaspoon oregano
½ pound lean ground beef	⅛ teaspoon pepper
⅓ cup tomato paste	1 small bay leaf
⅔ cup water	½ cup tomatoes, fresh or
2½ teaspoons Italian	canned
seasoning	2 cups cooked spaghetti,
½ teaspoon onion powder	drained
¼ teaspoon garlic powder	

STEPS IN PREPARATION:
1. Combine onion and ground beef.
2. Place in nonstick skillet and brown, draining off fat as it accumulates.
3. Add tomato paste, water, spices, herbs, and tomatoes.
4. Simmer 1 or more hours, adding more water if needed.
5. Serve ½ cup sauce over ½ cup cooked spaghetti.

STUFFED PEPPERS

Yield: 4 servings	**Each serving may be substituted**
Each serving: 1 stuffed pepper	**for:** 2 Bread
	2 Low-fat Meat

INGREDIENTS:

4 medium green peppers
½ pound lean ground beef
½ cup chopped onion
1 cup canned tomatoes, drained
1 cup cooked rice
½ teaspoon Italian seasoning

¼ teaspoon salt
Dash of pepper
1 tablespoon Worcestershire sauce
¼ cup bread crumbs
1 cup tomato sauce

STEPS IN PREPARATION:
1. Slice off stem end of peppers; remove seeds and membranes.
2. Blanch 5 to 10 minutes in boiling water.
3. Combine beef and onion in nonstick skillet.
4. Sauté over low heat until beef is browned; drain fat.
5. Add tomatoes; continue cooking until liquid is absorbed.
6. Remove from heat and stir in rice, Italian seasoning, salt, pepper, and Worcestershire sauce.
7. Place ½-cup portions of mixture into peppers; sprinkle breadcrumbs over mixture.
8. Place peppers in nonstick baking dish.
9. Bake at 350° about 20 minutes or until browned.
10. Heat sauce; pour ¼ cup over each pepper, and serve.

VEAL SCALLOPINI

Yield: 6 servings	**Each serving may be exchanged**
Each serving: ½ cup	**for:** 2 Medium-fat Meat
	1 Vegetable

INGREDIENTS:

½ cup chopped onion	1 cup tomato sauce
¼ cup chopped green	1 cup water
pepper	¼ teaspoon salt
1 tablespoon reduced-calorie	¼ teaspoon thyme
margarine	⅛ teaspoon pepper
1 pound veal cutlets, sliced	½ cup shredded low-fat
into thin strips	process American cheese

STEPS IN PREPARATION:

1. Sauté onion and green peppers in margarine in nonstick skillet; remove from skillet and set aside.
2. Place veal in skillet, and brown on both sides.
3. Add tomato sauce, water, salt, thyme, and pepper.
4. Return onions and green pepper to mixture.
5. Cover; simmer 15 minutes.
6. Remove from heat and sprinkle with cheese.

Note: Serve over rice, noodles, or spaghetti (count as a Bread Exchange).

BAKED PORK CHOPS WITH APPLE

Yield: 12 ounces pork	**Each serving may be exchanged**
Each Serving: 1 ounce	**for:** 1 Medium-fat Meat

INGREDIENTS:

4 pork chops, trimmed of fat	¼ teaspoon allspice
1 medium onion, sliced	Dash of pepper
½ cup fat-free chicken broth	1 medium apple, cut into
1 teaspoon dry mustard	¼-inch wedges
½ teaspoon salt	2 tablespoons parsley

STEPS IN PREPARATION:
1. Brown pork chops on both sides in nonstick skillet; drain fat from chops.
2. Place onion over chops.
3. Combine broth, mustard, salt, allspice, and pepper; mix well, pour over chops.
4. Heat to boiling; reduce heat.
5. Cover and simmer until pork is tender.
6. Arrange apple wedges over chops.
7. Cover, and cook about 4 minutes or until apple is tender.
8. Sprinkle with parsley.
9. Serve each serving with 1 to 2 apple wedges.

PORK CHOP DINNER

Yield: 7 servings	**Each serving may be exchanged**
Each serving: ⅓ cup rice with 1	**for:** 1 Bread
ounce pork	1 Medium-fat Meat

INGREDIENTS:

3 or 4 (½-inch thick) pork chops, trimmed of fat
¼ cup chopped onion
¼ cup chopped green pepper
1½ cups canned tomatoes

½ cup uncooked rice
1 teaspoon salt
¼ teaspoon dry mustard
⅛ teaspoon allspice
⅛ teaspoon pepper

STEPS IN PREPARATION:
1. Brown pork chops in nonstick skillet until tender.
2. Remove pork chops, and drain fat.
3. Sauté onion and green pepper in skillet until tender.
4. Combine tomatoes, uncooked rice, salt, mustard, allspice, and pepper; stir into sautéed mixture.
5. Place pork chops on top of mixture.
6. Cover; simmer 30 minutes or until rice is tender.

CREOLE PORK CHOPS

Yield: 4 servings **Each serving:** 2 ounces pork 　with sauce	**Each serving may be exchanged** **for:** 2 Medium-fat Meat 　2 Vegetable

INGREDIENTS:

4 pork chops, trimmed of fat ¼ cup chopped celery
1 (20-ounce) can tomatoes ½ teaspoon salt
⅓ cup chopped onion 1 bay leaf
¼ cup chopped green ¼ teaspoon oregano
　pepper ½ teaspoon liquid pepper

STEPS IN PREPARATION:

1. Brown chops in nonstick skillet.
2. Drain fat; add remaining ingredients.
3. Cover skillet; simmer for 1 hour or until chops are tender.
4. Divide sauce into 4 equal portions, and serve over pork.

HAM AND CHEESE CASSEROLE

Yield: 6 servings **Each serving:** 1/6th casserole	**Each serving may be exchanged** **for:** 1½ Bread 　2 Low-fat Meat 　1 Fat

INGREDIENTS:

6 slices bread, cubed ½ teaspoon dry mustard
1 cup grated low-fat process ½ teaspoon salt
　American cheese ½ teaspoon Worcestershire
1 cup chopped, cooked lean 　sauce
　ham 2 cups skim milk
3 eggs, beaten

STEPS IN PREPARATION:

1. Place bread cubes in nonstick 9- x 9-inch pan.
2. Sprinkle cheese on top of bread.

3. Place ham on top of cheese.
4. Combine beaten eggs with mustard, salt, Worcestershire sauce, and milk; beat well.
5. Pour over bread mixture.
6. Cover and refrigerate at least 6 hours.
7. Bake at 350° for 1 hour or until crust forms and mixture is firm enough to cut.
8. Cut into 6 equal portions and serve.

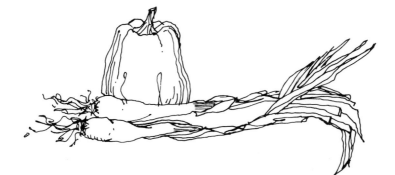

HAM SALAD

Yield: 7 servings	Each serving may be exchanged
Each serving: ⅓ cup	for: 1 Medium-fat Meat

INGREDIENTS:

2 cups ground lean cooked ham
½ cup minced green pepper
¼ cup finely minced green onions
4 teaspoons prepared mustard

½ cup reduced-calorie mayonnaise
2 tablespoons Worcestershire sauce
Pepper to taste
Lettuce leaves (optional)

STEPS IN PREPARATION:

1. Combine all ingredients in a mixing bowl.
2. Chill until ready to serve.
3. Serve on lettuce leaves, if desired.

HAM AND CORN CASSEROLE

Yield: 8 servings	**Each serving may be exchanged**
Each serving: ¾ cup	**for:** 1 Bread
	2 Medium-fat Meat
	1 Vegetable

INGREDIENTS:

3 tablespoons reduced-calorie margarine
3 tablespoons flour
1½ cups skim milk
½ teaspoon dry mustard
¼ teaspoon salt
⅛ teaspoon pepper
¼ teaspoon Worcestershire sauce

1 (20-ounce) can whole kernel corn, drained
¼ cup chopped onion
¼ cup chopped green pepper
2 cups cubed lean cooked ham
1 cup breadcrumbs
1 cup grated low-fat process American cheese

STEPS IN PREPARATION:

1. Make white sauce of margarine, flour, and milk (see page 167 for steps).
2. Stir in mustard, salt, pepper, and Worcestershire sauce.
3. Add corn, onion, green pepper, and ham.
4. Pour mixture into nonstick casserole.
5. Top with breadcrumbs and cheese.
6. Bake at 375° for 25 minutes or until bubbly, and serve.

Variety (organ) meats, lean meats, poultry, shellfish, egg yolk, green leafy vegetables, whole grain and enriched cereals and breads, legumes, nuts, and molasses provide iron.

BARBECUED FRANKS AND BEANS

Yield: 4 servings	**Each serving may be exchanged**
Each serving: 1 cup	**for:** 2 Bread
	1 High-fat Meat
	1 Fat

INGREDIENTS:

¾ cup chopped onion
1 tablespoon all-purpose
   flour
1 tablespoon vinegar
1 teaspoon Worcestershire
   sauce
Sugar substitute to equal 4
   teaspoons sugar
½ teaspoon chili powder

½ teaspoon salt
1 beef bouillon cube
½ cup boiling water
1 cup canned tomatoes,
   drained
2 cups canned kidney beans,
   drained
4 frankfurters, cut diagonally
   into chunks

STEPS IN PREPARATION:

1. Sauté onion in nonstick pan.
2. Blend flour, vinegar, Worcestershire sauce, sugar substitute, chili powder, and salt.
3. Quickly stir in onion.
4. Dissolve bouillon cube in boiling water and add to mixture.
5. Add tomatoes, kidney beans, and franks.
6. Simmer covered until heated thoroughly, and serve.

POULTRY

Poultry can be used in many dishes. It contains high-quality protein, and several vitamins and minerals, including niacin, iron, phosphorous, and magnesium. Chicken and turkey are low in fat, while duck and goose are higher in fat. The skin of all poultry should be removed before cooking to eliminate the layer of fat just underneath the skin. Chicken livers are an economical variety item which can be baked, stewed with onions and chicken broth, or mixed with other ingredients in casseroles.

Although there is generally a large proportion of bone to meat in poultry, it is often a good buy. For the best economy, compare the cost of fresh, frozen, or canned poultry, as well as the price of parts versus the cost of the whole bird. Consider the manner in which you will prepare and serve the poultry when deciding how to buy.

Chicken is available in different classes; size, age, and sex of the chicken determine class. A broiler or fryer is usually 10 to 16 weeks of age with smooth, thin, soft skin and tender meat with little fat under the skin. A roaster is usually under eight months of age with characteristics similar to a broiler or fryer but with more fat. A stewing chicken or hen is usually more than 10 months of age and has less tender, firm flesh and well-developed connective tissue, as well as more fat than younger birds. Any young bird may be chosen for roasting or grilling. Young birds or hens may be used for stewing or in casseroles, depending on cost per pound. Fat which accumulates during stewing should be skimmed as it accumulates. Poultry is cooked when the thigh joint moves freely.

Use fresh poultry within one to two days after purchase. Wash and pat dry before cooking. If frozen, always thaw in the refrigerator, not at room temperature. Do not refreeze once thawed.

CHICKEN AND DUMPLINGS

Yield: 6 servings	**Each serving may be exchanged**
Each serving: ¾ cup	**for:** 2 Medium-fat Meat
	1 Starch

INGREDIENTS:

1 small chicken (1½ pounds)   ½ stalk celery (¼ cup)
1½ cups water   ¼ cup onion
¼ teaspoon salt   Dumplings (recipe follows)

STEPS IN PREPARATION:

1. Disjoint chicken and remove skin; place in large pan.
2. Add water, salt, celery, and onion; simmer 1 to 2 hours or until meat is tender.
3. Remove chicken from bone; return chicken to chicken stock.
4. Bring chicken and stock to a boil; add rolled dumplings.
5. Cover and boil gently 8 to 10 minutes.

Dumplings:

INGREDIENTS:

1 cup all-purpose flour   3 tablespoons shortening
1 teaspoon baking powder   ¼ cup skim milk
½ teaspoon salt

STEPS IN PREPARATION:

1. Combine flour, baking powder, and salt.
2. Cut in shortening.
3. Add milk to make a stiff dough.
4. Roll dough out to about ⅛-inch thickness, and cut into 1-inch strips or squares.

To store meats and poultry, remove from grocery wrap and wrap loosely in waxed paper or foil.

BAKED CHICKEN BREASTS

Yield: 3 servings	**Each serving may be exchanged**
Each serving: 2 ounces	**for:** ½ Bread
	2 Low-fat Meat

INGREDIENTS:

½ teaspoon celery salt
½ teaspoon paprika
⅛ teaspoon pepper
Dash of garlic powder
½ cup plain low-fat yogurt
1 tablespoon lemon juice

1 teaspoon Worcestershire
   sauce
3 chicken breast halves, skin
   removed
¾ cup crushed corn flakes

STEPS IN PREPARATION:

1. Combine all ingredients except chicken and corn flakes; blend mixture well.
2. Spoon yogurt mixture over chicken to coat well.
3. Cover chicken, and refrigerate overnight.
4. Coat each chicken breast with corn flake crumbs.
5. Place chicken in shallow nonstick baking dish.
6. Bake at 350° for 45 to 60 minutes or until golden brown; baste once.

BAKED CHICKEN WITH RICE

Yield: 6 servings	**Each serving may be exchanged**
Each serving: 2 ounces chicken	**for:** 2 Bread
with ⅔ cup rice	2 Medium-fat Meat

INGREDIENTS:

1 cup uncooked rice
1 package onion soup mix,
   divided
6 chicken breast halves, skin
   removed

1 (10¾-ounce) can cream of
   mushroom soup
1½ cups water
⅛ teaspoon pepper

STEPS IN PREPARATION:
1. Spread rice evenly in bottom of 9- x 9- x 2-inch nonstick baking dish.
2. Sprinkle with ¼ onion soup mix.
3. Place chicken on top of rice.
4. Add remaining onion soup mix.
5. Combine mushroom soup, water, and pepper.
6. Pour soup mixture over chicken.
7. Cover with foil; bake at 325° for 2 hours.
8. Remove foil, and serve.

CREOLE CHICKEN

Yield: 4 servings	**Each serving may be exchanged**
Each serving: ½ small chicken breast with ⅓ cup sauce	**for:** 2 Low-fat Meat
	1 Vegetable
	1 Fat

INGREDIENTS:

2 small chicken breasts, halved, skin removed
½ cup chopped celery
⅓ cup sliced onion
1 medium green pepper, cut in strips
1 (16-ounce) can tomatoes
½ teaspoon salt
½ teaspoon thyme
⅛ teaspoon pepper

STEPS IN PREPARATION:
1. Place chicken breasts on broiler pan 5 inches from heating element.
2. Broil chicken 10 minutes or until browned, turning once.
3. Combine remaining ingredients in large nonstick skillet.
4. Bring mixture to a boil; cover, and cook over medium heat 10 minutes.
5. Add chicken; cover and reduce heat.
6. Simmer 30 minutes or until tender, and serve.

HERBED CHICKEN

Yield: 6 servings Each serving: ½ small chicken breast	Each serving may be exchanged for: 2 Low-fat Meat

INGREDIENTS:

3 small chicken breasts,
  halved, skin removed
½ teaspoon salt
2 teaspoons dried rosemary

¼ teaspoon pepper
2 chicken bouillon cubes
1 cup water

STEPS IN PREPARATION:
1. Place chicken in nonstick baking dish.
2. Season with salt, rosemary, and pepper.
3. Crumble bouillon cubes between pieces of chicken.
4. Add water, pouring into a corner of pan.
5. Cover with foil; bake at 350° for 1 hour.
6. Uncover and baste with drippings.
7. Brown under the broiler before serving.

SOY CHICKEN

Yield: 6 servings Each serving: 2 ounces	Each serving may be exchanged for: 2 Low-fat Meat

INGREDIENTS:

6 chicken breast halves, skin
  removed
Dash of onion powder
Dash of garlic powder

⅓ cup soy sauce
⅓ cup Worcestershire sauce
⅓ cup vinegar
⅓ cup water

STEPS IN PREPARATION:
1. Sprinkle both sides of chicken with onion and garlic
   powders.
2. Place chicken in 2-inch-deep baking dish.

3. Combine soy sauce, Worcestershire sauce, vinegar, and water.
4. Pour sauce over chicken.
5. Cover and refrigerate several hours or overnight.
6. Bake, uncovered, at 350° for 1 hour or until tender.

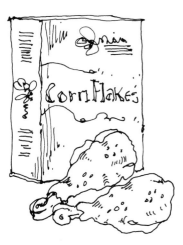

OVEN-FRIED CHICKEN

Yield: 4 servings	**Each serving may be exchanged**
Each serving: 2 ounces	**for:** ½ Bread
	2 Low-fat Meat

INGREDIENTS:

4 small chicken breasts (or 8 small legs or thighs)
1 cup crushed corn flakes
¼ teaspoon paprika

¼ teaspoon onion powder
¼ teaspoon garlic powder
¼ teaspoon curry powder
4 teaspoons skim milk

STEPS IN PREPARATION:

1. Remove skin from chicken.
2. Combine crushed corn flakes, paprika, and powders.
3. Roll chicken in milk.
4. Roll chicken in corn flake mixture.
5. Place chicken in small nonstick baking dish.
6. Bake at 350° for 20 to 30 minutes or until golden brown.

CHICKEN AND VEGETABLE CASSEROLE

Yield: 4 servings
Each serving: 1 cup

Each serving may be exchanged for: ½ Bread
2 Medium-fat Meat
1 Vegetable

INGREDIENTS:

1 (10¾-ounce) can cream of
mushroom soup
¼ cup skim milk
1 teaspoon Worcestershire
sauce
1 cup diced, cooked chicken
(no skin)

1 cup cooked sliced okra
¼ cup chopped celery
¼ cup chopped green
pepper

STEPS IN PREPARATION:

1. Combine soup, milk, and Worcestershire sauce.
2. Add chicken, okra, celery, and green pepper.
3. Pour into nonstick 1-quart casserole.
4. Bake at 350° for 20 minutes.

CHICKEN AND RICE CASSEROLE

Yield: 6 servings
Each serving: ½ cup

Each serving may be exchanged for: 1 Bread
2 Medium-fat Meat

INGREDIENTS:

2 hard-cooked eggs,
chopped
1 (10¾-ounce) can cream of
mushroom soup
1 small onion, chopped
1½ cups diced, cooked
chicken (no skin)
1 cup cooked rice

½ cup chopped celery
¼ cup reduced-calorie
mayonnaise
1 tablespoon lemon juice
¼ cup soft bread crumbs
1 tablespoon dry butter
substitute

STEPS IN PREPARATION:
1. Combine eggs, soup, onion, chicken, rice, celery, mayonnaise, and lemon juice, stirring well.
2. Spoon mixture into shallow nonstick 2-quart casserole.
3. Combine bread crumbs and butter substitute; sprinkle over top of casserole.
4. Bake at 350°, uncovered, for 40 to 45 minutes or until bubbly.

CHICKEN SALAD

Yield: 6 servings	**Each serving may be exchanged**
Each serving: ¾ cup	**for:** 2 Low-fat Meat
	1 Fat

INGREDIENTS:

2 cups diced, cooked chicken (no skin)
1 cup finely chopped celery
⅔ cup chopped onion
¾ cup reduced-calorie mayonnaise
1 tablespoon chopped pimiento

1 teaspoon salt
¼ teaspoon pepper
1 teaspoon Worcestershire sauce
Lettuce leaves (optional)

STEPS IN PREPARATION:
1. Combine all ingredients; mix well.
2. Cover; refrigerate until ready to serve.
3. Serve on lettuce leaves, if desired.

Keep celery fresh and crisp by wrapping in paper towels; place in plastic bag in refrigerator. The towels absorb excess moisture.

CHICKEN LIVERS

Yield: 5 servings	Each serving may be exchanged
Each serving: 2 ounces	for: 2 Medium-fat Meat

INGREDIENTS:

1 pound chicken livers	½ cup dry white wine
¾ teaspoon salt	1 tablespoon Worcestershire
¼ teaspoon pepper	sauce
3 tablespoons	
reduced-calorie	
margarine	

STEPS IN PREPARATION:
1. Wash and drain livers; sprinkle with salt and pepper.
2. Place livers in nonstick skillet; sauté in margarine until brown.
3. Combine wine and Worcestershire sauce; pour over livers.
4. Cover tightly and simmer 30 minutes.

CHICKEN LIVERS AND RICE

Yield: 8 servings	Each serving may be exchanged
Each serving: ½ cup	for: 1 Bread
	1 Medium-fat Meat

INGREDIENTS:

2 teaspoons reduced-calorie	2 tablespoons
margarine	reduced-calorie
3 tablespoons minced onion	margarine
2 cups cooked rice	1 (10¾-ounce) can cream of
½ pound chicken livers, cut	chicken soup
into 1-inch pieces	½ cup skim milk
2 tablespoons all-purpose	1 tablespoon chopped
flour	parsley
	Dash of pepper

STEPS IN PREPARATION:
1. Melt 2 teaspoons margarine in non-stick saucepan.
2. Add onion, and cook until tender.
3. Combine onion and rice; set aside.
4. Dredge chicken livers lightly in flour.
5. Sauté livers in 2 tablespoons margarine in nonstick skillet until browned on each side.
6. Combine livers, rice mixture, and remaining ingredients.
7. Place in nonstick 1½-quart casserole.
8. Bake at 375° for 30 minutes until hot and bubbly.

TURKEY HASH

Yield: 6 servings **Each serving:** ½ cup	**Each serving may be exchanged for:** 1 Bread 1 Medium-fat Meat

INGREDIENTS:

¼ cup chopped onion
2 teaspoons reduced-calorie margarine
1 cup diced, cooked turkey (no skin)
1 (10¾-ounce) can cream of celery soup

1½ cups cooked diced potatoes
⅔ cup cooked green peas
¼ cup shredded low-fat process American cheese
Paprika

STEPS IN PREPARATION:
1. Sauté onion in margarine in nonstick skillet until tender.
2. Add turkey, soup, potatoes, and peas.
3. Place mixture in 1-quart nonstick casserole.
4. Top with shredded cheese and paprika.
5. Bake at 350° for 30 minutes.

Plan ahead for times when meals may not be readily available. Carry ("brown-bag") foods that will not spoil but will fit into your meal plan.

RICE
AND PASTA

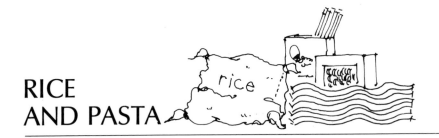

Rice and pasta are popular foods which are grain products; both add carbohydrate and some protein to the diet. If unmilled or enriched, they are good sources of vitamins and iron. Unmilled rice is also a good source of fiber.

Rice is available in short- and long-grain varieties. Short-grain rice cooks tender and moist, and the grains tend to cling together. It is usually favored for croquettes, pudding, or rice rings, where a molding quality is desired. Long-grain rice is fluffy, and the grains separate after cooking; it is preferred for serving with stews and creamed foods.

Rice is available in several forms. Pre-cooked rice is completely cooked and requires only steaming in boiling water. Converted rice is parboiled before milling to retain most of its nutrients. Regular or polished rice is cleaned, washed, and graded during the milling process and has had the bran layer removed; thus the fiber and most nutrients have also been removed. Enriched rice has had vitamins and minerals added to it.

Brown rice is often preferred to white rice because it is whole-grain rice with all nutrients and fiber intact. Wild rice is not a real rice but is the seed of marsh grass.

Rice can be served hot or cold as a breakfast cereal, as a meal accompaniment, or in main-dish casseroles, salads, and desserts.

Pasta also has a wide variety of uses and comes in hundreds of forms and shapes. Good pasta is made from semolina flour milled from durum wheat. Pasta products such as macaroni, noodles, and spaghetti are generally enriched and provide B vitamins and iron. Egg noodles have egg yolks added in preparation.

Various sauces may be added to pasta to make meat, vegetable, or fish meals. For variety and economy, use pasta with leftovers.

BAKED RICE

Yield: 9 servings	Each serving may be exchanged
Each serving: ⅓ cup	for: 1 Bread

INGREDIENTS:

1 cup uncooked rice
1 (10½-ounce) can beef
   consommé

1 (10½-ounce) can onion
   soup in beef stock

STEPS IN PREPARATION:
1. Place rice in nonstick 1-quart casserole.
2. Pour consommé and soup over rice.
3. Stir enough to mix.
4. Cover casserole with foil.
5. Bake at 350° for 1 hour; stir occasionally.

BLACK-EYED PEAS WITH RICE

Yield: 9 servings	Each serving may be exchanged
Each serving: ⅓ cup	for: 1 Bread

INGREDIENTS:

½ cup chopped onion
2 teaspoons reduced-calorie
   margarine
1 (15-ounce) can black-eyed
   peas, drained

1 (14½-ounce) can stewed
   tomatoes, undrained
⅔ cup cooked rice
¼ teaspoon salt
¼ teaspoon pepper

STEPS IN PREPARATION:
1. Sauté onion in margarine in nonstick skillet until tender.
2. Add remaining ingredients and stir well.
3. Spoon mixture into nonstick 1-quart casserole.
4. Bake at 350° for 30 minutes.

For fluffy rice, cook in pan with lid on and
do not stir while cooking.

HOLIDAY RICE

Yield: 9 servings	**Each serving may be exchanged**
Each serving: ½ cup	**for:** 1 Bread

INGREDIENTS:

½ cup chopped onion
½ cup chopped celery
½ cup chopped green
    pepper
2 tablespoons
    reduced-calorie
    margarine

2½ cups cooked rice
1 cup cooked chopped
    broccoli
1 teaspoon salt
2 tablespoons chopped
    parsley
Fresh parsley sprigs
    (optional)

STEPS IN PREPARATION:

1. Combine onion, celery, and green pepper; sauté mixture in margarine in nonstick skillet.
2. Add rice, broccoli, salt, and parsley; stir well.
3. Pour into warm nonstick 5-cup ring mold, and turn out onto serving platter.
4. Garnish with sprigs of parsley before serving, if desired.

BAKED CHEESE AND RICE

Yield: 7 servings	**Each serving may be exchanged**
Each serving: ⅓ cup	**for:** 1 Bread
	½ Low-fat Meat

INGREDIENTS:

¾ cup skim milk
1 cup grated low-fat process
    American cheese
¼ teaspoon salt
Dash of pepper
1 teaspoon reduced-calorie
    margarine

½ teaspoon Worcestershire
    sauce
2 cups cooked rice
Dash of paprika

STEPS IN PREPARATION:
1. Combine milk and cheese in nonstick saucepan; cook over low heat, stirring constantly, until cheese melts.
2. Add salt, pepper, margarine, and Worcestershire sauce; blend well.
3. Add rice, and mix lightly.
4. Turn into nonstick 1-quart baking dish; sprinkle with paprika.
5. Bake at 350° for 15 minutes or until lightly browned.

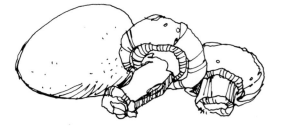

PARTY RICE

Yield: 6 servings	**Each serving may be exchanged**
Each serving: ½ cup	**for:** 1 Bread
	1 Medium-fat Meat
	1 Fat

INGREDIENTS:
1 cup cooked rice
1 cup diced mushrooms
1 cup cream of mushroom soup, undiluted
1 cup grated low-fat process American cheese
1 egg, beaten
1 (4-ounce) jar pimiento, drained and chopped
½ cup pecans or almonds, chopped
Fresh parsley (optional)

STEPS IN PREPARATION:
1. Combine all ingredients except parsley in mixing bowl.
2. Place in 1-quart nonstick baking dish.
3. Cover and bake at 350° for 30 minutes.
4. Garnish with fresh parsley before serving, if desired.

MEXICAN RICE

| **Yield:** 10 servings | **Each serving may be exchanged** |
| **Each serving:** ⅓ cup | **for:** 1 Bread |

INGREDIENTS:

⅔ cup chopped onion
1 tablespoon reduced-calorie
   margarine
1 cup uncooked rice
1 cup chopped green
   pepper

1 (8-ounce) can whole
   tomatoes, chopped
1 teaspoon salt
1 teaspoon chili powder
2 cups water

STEPS IN PREPARATION:

1. Sauté onion in margarine in nonstick skillet until tender.
2. Stir in rice, green pepper, tomatoes, salt, and chili powder.
3. Add water.
4. Bring to boil; reduce heat and simmer covered for 20
   minutes or until liquid is absorbed and rice is cooked.

HAM "FRIED" RICE

Yield: 7 servings	**Each serving may be exchanged**
Each serving: ¾ cup	**for:** 1 Bread
	1 Medium-fat Meat

INGREDIENTS:

½ cup chopped onions
1 cup chopped celery
½ cup chopped green
   pepper
1 tablespoon reduced-calorie
   margarine
1½ cups diced, cooked lean
   ham

½ teaspoon seasoned salt
Dash of garlic powder
½ to 1 teaspoon curry
   powder, to taste
2 cups cooked rice

STEPS IN PREPARATION:
1. Sauté onion, celery, and green pepper in margarine in large nonstick skillet.
2. Add ham, seasoned salt, and garlic powder.
3. Stir to blend, but do not cook.
4. Add curry powder to taste.
5. Add rice to mixture.
6. Heat to warm before serving.

HAM GRITS

Yield: 11 servings	**Each serving may be exchanged**
Each serving: ¼ cup	**for:** 1 Bread
	½ Low-fat Meat

INGREDIENTS:

1 cup grits, uncooked
½ cup chopped onion
1 medium green pepper, chopped
2 teaspoons reduced-calorie margarine

1 cup ground, cooked lean ham
3 medium tomatoes, chopped

STEPS IN PREPARATION:
1. Cook grits according to directions on package.
2. Brown onion and green pepper in margarine in nonstick skillet.
3. Add ham and tomatoes.
4. Cook over medium heat until liquid evaporates.
5. Add cooked grits to ham mixture; mix well.
6. Place in nonstick 1-quart casserole.
7. Bake at 375° for 30 to 45 minutes.

No one food provides all nutrients; to get all nutrients you need, eat a variety of foods every day.

NOODLES WITH "BUTTER" SAUCE

Yield: 9 servings	**Each serving may be exchanged**
Each serving: ⅓ cup	**for:** 1 Bread
	1 Fat

INGREDIENTS:

1 6-ounce package medium egg noodles.
¼ cup reduced-calorie margarine, melted
Dash of garlic powder

2 tablespoons chopped fresh parsley
2 tablespoons grated Parmesan cheese

STEPS IN PREPARATION:

1. Cook noodles according to package directions; drain well.
2. Pour margarine over noodles.
3. Add garlic powder and parsley; toss gently to mix.
4. Place noodle mixture in serving dish.
5. Sprinkle with cheese and serve.

NOODLE AND RICE CASSEROLE

Yield: 18 servings	**Each serving may be exchanged**
Each serving: ¼ cup	**for:** 1 Bread
	1 Fat

INGREDIENTS:

1 (4-ounce) package fine noodles
2 tablespoons reduced-calorie margarine
1 cup uncooked rice

1 cup fat-free chicken stock
1 (10½-ounce) can onion soup
2 tablespoons soy sauce
½ cup sliced and toasted almonds

STEPS IN PREPARATION:

1. Brown uncooked noodles in margarine in nonstick skillet until just golden.

2. Add rice, chicken stock, onion soup, and soy sauce.
3. Cover; simmer 30 minutes or until rice is done.
4. Turn into nonstick 2-quart casserole; sprinkle with almonds.
5. Bake, uncovered, at 325° for 30 minutes.

VERMICELLI WITH TOMATO SAUCE

Yield: 6 servings	**Each serving may be exchanged**
Each serving: ½ cup vermicelli	**for:** 1 Bread
with ½ cup sauce	1 Vegetable

INGREDIENTS:

½ cup chopped onion
1 teaspoon reduced-calorie margarine
3 cups peeled, chopped tomatoes
1 teaspoon paprika
½ teaspoon salt

½ teaspoon dried whole basil
½ teaspoon dried whole oregano
⅛ teaspoon pepper
3 cups hot cooked, and drained vermicelli

STEPS IN PREPARATION:

1. Sauté onion in margarine in nonstick skillet.
2. Add tomatoes, paprika, salt, basil, oregano, and pepper; cover and simmer 5 minutes, stirring occasionally.
3. Remove from heat, and serve over hot vermicelli.

SALADS AND
SALAD DRESSINGS

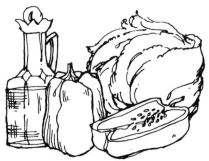

Salads have many uses in a diabetic diet; they can be served as main dishes, meal accompaniments, appetizers, and desserts. The ingredients used in a salad generally determine how it will be served. Prepared with selected ingredients, salads can be low in calories and high in nutritional value.

Left over meats, poultry, or fish make excellent main-dish salads, and vegetable salads can be used as side dishes. Green salads are low in calories and add color and texture to meals. A congealed vegetable salad is often a good choice for variety, or choose a salad such as potato or macaroni which is higher in carbohydrates and thus caloric content.

Fruit salads are generally low in calories but high in nutrients, such as vitamins, minerals, and fiber. Select fruits based on the use of the fruit. When fruit is used whole or in large pieces, select top-quality fruits; when fruit is to be cut into small pieces, appearance need not be perfect. Be sure to select fresh fruits, water-packed canned fruits, or frozen unsweetened fruits.

To complete the salad, select a dressing that will complement the flavor of the ingredients. Some salad dressings will be "free" in measured amounts; some will count as Fat Exchanges.

PICKLED BEET SALAD

Yield: 6 servings	Each serving may be exchanged
Each serving: ½ cup	for: 1 Vegetable

INGREDIENTS:

2 cups canned beets with
    juice
¼ cup vinegar
½ teaspoon salt
¼ teaspoon cinnamon

⅛ teaspoon cloves
Sugar substitute to equal 2
    tablespoons sugar
Dash of pepper

STEPS IN PREPARATION:

1. Drain beets and place in medium bowl; reserve juice in a saucepan.
2. Add remaining ingredients to beet juice.
3. Bring juice to boil; immediately remove from heat.
4. Pour juice mixture over beets.
5. Chill; drain beets before serving.

"CREAMY" SLICED CUCUMBER SALAD

Yield: 5 servings	Each serving may be exchanged
Each serving: ½ cup	for: 1 Vegetable

INGREDIENTS:

2 medium cucumbers
½ teaspoon salt
1 (8-ounce) carton plain
    low-fat yogurt

¼ teaspoon dillweed
2 tablespoons minced onion
1 tablespoon lemon juice

STEPS IN PREPARATION:

1. Peel cucumbers and slice.
2. Spread slices in large shallow pan.
3. Sprinkle with salt, and let stand 15 minutes; drain well.
4. Combine remaining ingredients in medium bowl; mix well.
5. Add cucumber slices; mix well before serving.

COLE SLAW

| Yield: 8 servings | Each serving may be exchanged |
| Each serving: ½ cup | for: 1 Vegetable |

INGREDIENTS:

4 cups shredded cabbage
½ cup shredded carrots
⅓ cup reduced-calorie
  mayonnaise

2 tablespoons prepared
  mustard
½ teaspoon salt
2 tablespoons vinegar

STEPS IN PREPARATION:
1. Combine all ingredients.
2. Toss lightly, and serve.

POTATO SALAD

Yield: 4 servings	Each serving may be exchanged
Each serving: ½ cup	for: 1 Bread
	½ Medium-fat meat

INGREDIENTS:

2 hard-cooked eggs,
  chopped
2 medium potatoes, cooked
  and diced
2 tablespoons diced celery
2 teaspoons chopped onion
2 teaspoons chopped green
  pepper
2 teaspoons chopped
  pimiento

2 teaspoons chopped dill
  pickle
2 tablespoons prepared
  mustard
2 tablespoons
  reduced-calorie
  mayonnaise

STEPS IN PREPARATION:
1. Combine all ingredients.
2. Refrigerate until served.

TOMATO ASPIC

Yield: 7 servings	**Each serving may be exchanged**
Each serving: ½ cup	**for:** 1 Vegetable

INGREDIENTS:

3 cups tomato juice	2 envelopes unflavored
1 stalk celery, sliced	gelatin
1 small onion, sliced	⅔ cup chilled tomato juice
2 lemon slices	¼ cup vinegar
1 small bay leaf	¼ cup finely chopped celery
1 teaspoon salt	Lettuce leaves (optional)
⅛ teaspoon pepper	

STEPS IN PREPARATION:

1. Combine 3 cups tomato juice, celery, onion, lemon, bay leaf, salt, and pepper.
2. Simmer, uncovered, for 10 minutes; strain mixture, and remove bay leaf. Set aside.
3. Sprinkle gelatin over chilled tomato juice and vinegar to soften.
4. Add hot strained juice to gelatin, stirring until gelatin dissolves.
5. Refrigerate until mixture begins to thicken.
6. Add chopped celery; stir.
7. Pour into 7 (½-cup) molds; chill until firm.
8. Unmold and serve on lettuce leaves, if desired.

Wash most vegetables; trim any wilted parts or excess leaves before storing in crisper compartment of refrigerator. Keep potatoes and onions in a cool, dark place with plenty of air circulation to prevent sprouting.

MARINATED VEGETABLE SALAD

Yield: 10 servings	**Each serving may be exchanged**
Each serving: ½ cup	**for**: 1 Vegetable

INGREDIENTS:

3 cups carrots, sliced diagonally	1 teaspoon celery seeds
1 cup chopped celery	½ cup reduced-calorie Italian salad dressing
½ cup chopped green pepper	¼ cup vinegar
1 medium onion, thinly sliced	¼ cup water
	Sugar substitute to equal 1 cup sugar

STEPS IN PREPARATION:
1. Place carrots in small saucepan; cover with water, and boil about 10 minutes or until crisp-tender; drain well.
2. Place carrots, celery, green pepper, onion, and celery seeds in large shallow dish; toss lightly and set aside.
3. Combine remaining ingredients in small saucepan, mixing well; bring to a boil, stirring often.
4. Pour sauce mixture over vegetables.
5. Cover and chill overnight.

MACARONI SALAD

Yield: 7 servings	**Each serving may be exchanged**
Each serving: ½ cup	**for**: 1½ Bread
	1 Fat

INGREDIENTS:

3 cups hot cooked macaroni, drained	1 tablespoon minced onion
⅓ cup chopped celery	2 tablespoons minced fresh parsley
2 hard-cooked eggs, diced	½ teaspoon salt
⅓ cup reduced-calorie mayonnaise	¼ teaspoon paprika

STEPS IN PREPARATION:
1. Combine all ingredients in large bowl.
2. Mix well.
3. Cover and refrigerate until served.

Note: Flavor is best when ingredients are allowed to blend several hours or overnight.

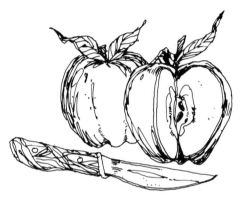

SPICED APPLE RINGS

Yield: 12 servings	**Each serving may be exchanged**
Each serving: ½ cup	**for:** 1 Fruit

INGREDIENTS:
6 medium firm apples
Sugar substitute to equal 1½ cups sugar
2 sticks cinnamon
2 to 3 whole cloves
1½ cups unsweetened cranberry juice
¼ cup lemon juice

STEPS IN PREPARATION:
1. Wash and core apples; slice unpeeled into thick slices.
2. Place in flat pan.
3. Combine remaining ingredients, and boil 5 minutes.
4. Reserve ¼ cup juice mixture, and set aside.
5. Pour remaining juice mixture over apple slices.
6. Bake at 350° for 45 minutes or until apple slices appear transparent; baste occasionally with the ¼ cup juice mixture. Serve hot or cold as a salad.

APPLE SALAD

Yield: 8 servings	**Each serving may be exchanged**
Each serving: ¼ cup	**for:** 1 Fruit

INGREDIENTS:

2 apples, diced and unpared
½ cup diced celery
¼ cup raisins
1 tablespoon lemon juice

1 tablespoon reduced-calorie
  mayonnaise
Lettuce leaves (optional)

STEPS IN PREPARATION:
1. Combine all ingredients except lettuce; mix well.
2. Refrigerate until served.
3. Serve on lettuce leaves, if desired.

CARROT-PINEAPPLE GELATIN SALAD

Yield: 6 servings	**Each serving may be exchanged**
Each serving: ½ cup	**for:** 1 Vegetable

INGREDIENTS:

1 envelope unflavored
  gelatin
½ cup cold unsweetened
  orange juice
1 cup boiling water
Sugar substitute to equal 3
  tablespoons sugar

⅛ teaspoon salt
3 tablespoons lemon juice
½ cup shredded carrots
½ cup unsweetened canned
  crushed pineapple,
  drained
Lettuce leaves (optional)

STEPS IN PREPARATION:
1. Sprinkle gelatin into cold orange juice to soften.
2. Add softened gelatin to boiling water, and stir until
   thoroughly dissolved.
3. Add sugar substitute, salt, and lemon juice.
4. Chill until slightly thickened; fold in carrots and pineapple.
5. Turn into large (3-cup) mold, or 6 individual molds.
6. Chill until firm.
7. Unmold and serve on lettuce leaf, if desired.

CARROT-RAISIN SALAD

Yield: 7 servings	**Each serving may be exchanged**
Each serving: ½ cup	**for:** 1 Fruit
	1 Vegetable

INGREDIENTS:

2 cups grated carrots
1 cup unsweetened crushed
   pineapple, drained
½ cup raisins

1 (8-ounce) carton plain
   low-fat yogurt
7 lettuce leaves (optional)

STEPS IN PREPARATION:
1. Combine carrots, pineapple, and raisins; mix well.
2. Chill for 2 to 3 hours.
3. Stir in yogurt, and serve on lettuce leaf, if desired.

PINEAPPLE-ORANGE SALAD

Yield: 12 servings	**Each serving may be exchanged**
Each serving: ¼ cup	**for:** 1 Fruit

INGREDIENTS:

2 cups unsweetened orange
   juice, divided
2 envelopes unflavored
   gelatin
2 cups unsweetened,
   crushed pineapple,
   drained

Sugar substitute to equal ¼
   cup sugar
¼ teaspoon salt
2 tablespoons lemon juice
½ teaspoon almond extract

STEPS IN PREPARATION:
1. Pour ½ cup orange juice into a large bowl.
2. Sprinkle gelatin over juice and allow to soften.
3. Heat the remaining 1½ cups orange juice, and pour over softened gelatin mixture; blend well.
4. Add remaining ingredients; mix well.
5. Pour into 3-cup mold and refrigerate until set.
6. Unmold and serve.

PEACH-GINGER ALE MOLD

Yield: 8 servings **Each serving:** 1 cup	**Each serving may be exchanged** **for:** 1 Fruit ½ Fat

INGREDIENTS:

1 (16-ounce) can
  unsweetened peach
  slices
2 (3-ounce) packages dietetic
  orange or lemon gelatin

1½ cups boiling water
1 (12-ounce) can diet ginger
  ale
¼ cup chopped walnuts

STEPS IN PREPARATION:
1. Drain peaches; set aside ½ cup peach slices.
2. Arrange remaining peaches in bottom of 1½-quart mold, overlapping slices.
3. Dissolve gelatin in boiling water; add ginger ale, and chill until slightly thickened.
4. Beat until fluffy.
5. Chop reserved ½ cup peach slices, and fold into gelatin along with walnuts.
6. Spoon gelatin mixture over peaches in mold.
7. Refrigerate until served; unmold and serve.

STRAWBERRY DELIGHT SALAD

Yield: 4 servings **Each serving:** ½ cup	**Each serving may be exchanged** **for:** 1 Fruit

INGREDIENTS:

1 (3-ounce) package dietetic
  strawberry gelatin
¾ cup chopped fresh
  strawberries
1 cup plain low-fat yogurt

1 teaspoon vanilla extract
Sugar substitute to equal 2
  teaspoons sugar

STEPS IN PREPARATION:
1. Prepare gelatin according to package directions.
2. Chill until slightly thickened.
3. Crush strawberries in blender or by hand; add to gelatin mixture.
4. Add yogurt, vanilla, and sugar substitute; stir mixture until well blended.
5. Pour into 4 individual molds; chill until set.
6. Unmold and serve.

FRESH FRUIT SALAD

Yield: 6 servings **Each serving:** ½ cup	**Each serving may be exchanged** **for:** 1 Fruit 1 Fat

INGREDIENTS:

½ small cantaloupe, pared and diced
½ cup sliced fresh strawberries
½ cup seedless green grapes, halved
¼ cup plain low-fat yogurt
2 tablespoons reduced-calorie mayonnaise

Brown sugar substitute to equal 1 tablespoon brown sugar
1 tablespoon chopped walnuts
6 lettuce leaves (optional)

STEPS IN PREPARATION:
1. Combine cantaloupe, strawberries, and grapes.
2. Combine yogurt, mayonnaise, brown sugar substitute, and nuts; mix well.
3. Stir yogurt mixture into fruit mixture.
4. Serve on lettuce leaves, if desired.

GELATIN FRUIT SALAD

Yield: 6 servings **Each serving:** 1/6th recipe	**Each serving may be exchanged** **for**: 1 Fruit

INGREDIENTS:

1 cup unsweetened
   applesauce
2 packages dietetic cherry
   gelatin
	1 cup diet ginger ale
	1 cup unsweetened crushed
	   pineapple, undrained

STEPS IN PREPARATION:
1. Heat applesauce to boiling; remove from heat.
2. Stir gelatin into applesauce; add ginger ale.
3. Chill until slightly set.
4. Stir in pineapple.
5. Pour into 8- x 8- x 2-inch pan or pour ¾ cup mixture into 6 individual molds; chill until set.
6. Cut into 6 equal portions or unmold individual molds and serve.

MIXED FRUIT SALAD

Yield: 16 servings **Each serving:** ¼ cup	**Each serving may be exchanged** **for**: 1 Fruit

INGREDIENTS:

1 cup chopped apples
1 cup sliced banana
1 (8-ounce) can
   unsweetened pineapple
   chunks, drained
½ cup raisins
	½ cup chopped celery
	⅓ cup reduced-calorie
	   mayonnaise
	1 tablespoon lemon juice
	Lettuce leaves (optional)

STEPS IN PREPARATION:
1. Combine all ingredients except lettuce leaves.
2. Toss gently to coat, and chill 1 to 2 hours.
3. Serve on lettuce leaves, if desired.

HERB DRESSING

Yield: ¾ cup	Free food
Each serving: 2 tablespoons	(Up to 2 servings per day)

INGREDIENTS:

½ cup wine vinegar
¼ cup salad vinegar
1 teaspoon onion powder

½ teaspoon garlic powder
1 teaspoon salad herbs
1 teaspoon fresh lemon juice

STEPS IN PREPARATION:
1. Combine all ingredients.
2. Refrigerate.
3. Shake well before using.

Note: This dressing may be kept for several weeks refrigerated in a closed container.

VINEGAR SALAD DRESSING

Yield: 1 cup	Free food
Each serving: 2 tablespoons	(Up to 3 servings per day)

INGREDIENTS:

1 cup apple vinegar
2 tablespoons lemon juice
2 teaspoons finely chopped
   onion

Sugar substitute to equal 4
   teaspoons sugar
½ teaspoon salt
½ teaspoon dry mustard
1 teaspoon paprika

STEPS IN PREPARATION:
1. Combine all ingredients.
2. Refrigerate.
3. Shake well before using.

Note: This dressing may be kept for several weeks refrigerated in a closed container.

ZERO SALAD DRESSING

Yield: ½ cup	Free food
Each serving: 2 tablespoons	(Up to 2 servings per day)

INGREDIENTS:

½ cup tomato juice
2 tablespoons lemon juice or
  vinegar
1 tablespoon minced onion
⅛ teaspoon salt

⅛ teaspoon oregano
Dash of pepper
Dash of garlic powder
  (optional)

STEPS IN PREPARATION:
1. Combine all ingredients in jar with tightly fitted top.
2. Refrigerate several hours.
3. Shake well before using.

Note: This dressing may be kept for several weeks refrigerated in a closed container.

CREAMY COTTAGE CHEESE-HERB DRESSING

Yield: 1⅓ cups	Free food
Each serving: 1 tablespoon	(Up to 2 servings per day)

INGREDIENTS:

1 cup low-fat cottage cheese
⅓ cup buttermilk

½ to 1 teaspoon dry
  dillweed

STEPS IN PREPARATION:
1. Place all ingredients in blender.
2. Process on medium speed until smooth and creamy.
3. Refrigerate until served.

Note: For variety, add herbs, spices, chopped dill pickles, dry mustard, liquid pepper, or onion powder to taste.

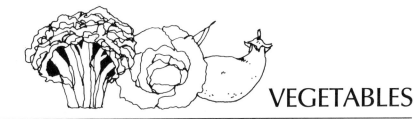

VEGETABLES

Vegetables make an excellent addition to a meal; they can be prepared in many ways to add flavor, color, texture, and variety. Generally, they are low in fat and calories but high in nutrient value, especially carbohydrates, vitamins, minerals, and fiber. Most dark green and dark yellow or orange vegetables are good sources of vitamins A and C. Include one excellent vitamin A source in your diet every other day and a vitamin C source daily. Vegetables rich in vitamin A include broccoli, spinach, mustard and turnip greens, carrots, sweet potatoes, and winter squash. Vegetables high in vitamin C include raw cabbage, tomatoes, green pepper, and salad greens. When cooked, however, vegetables lose most of their vitamin C.

Some vegetables (dried beans and peas, for example) are good sources of protein and the B vitamins, thiamin and niacin. Most vegetables are good sources of fiber, depending on the part of the plant eaten. Potatoes, for example, have little fiber without the skin, compared to stalk vegetables, such as celery, or leaf vegetables, such as lettuce or greens.

Fresh vegetables in season are excellent choices for nutritive value, flavor, and economy. When buying vegetables, look for freshness and crispness, and select those without bruises or soft spots. Most fresh vegetables should be stored in your refrigerator in plastic bags or covered containers to retain crispness and quality. Eggplant, onions, potatoes, winter squash, and sweet potatoes should be stored at room temperature or in a cool, dry, dark place.

This section contains some frequently used vegetables prepared in a variety of ways with the proper Exchanges to use in planning meals.

ASPARAGUS WITH HOT BACON DRESSING

Yield: 4 servings	**Each serving may be exchanged**
Each serving: ½ cup	**for:** 1 Vegetable
	½ Fat

INGREDIENTS:

2 medium slices bacon,
   finely diced
½ medium onion, finely
   chopped
¼ cup vinegar
¼ cup water

¼ teaspoon salt
Sugar substitute to equal 2
   teaspoons sugar
1 (14½-ounce) can
   asparagus, heated

STEPS IN PREPARATION:

1. Brown bacon in skillet until crisp.
2. Add onion and cook until tender; drain fat.
3. Add vinegar, water, and salt; bring to a boil.
4. Remove from heat, and add sugar substitute.
5. Pour dressing over hot asparagus, and serve.

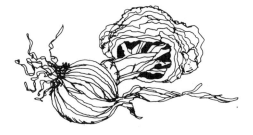

PICKLED BEETS

Yield: 6 servings	**Each serving may be exchanged**
Each serving: ½ cup	**for:** 1 Vegetable

INGREDIENTS:

1¾ cups sliced beets,
   drained
½ cup vinegar
6 whole cloves

Sugar substitute to equal 3
   tablespoons sugar
1 slice lemon
1 small onion, thinly sliced

STEPS IN PREPARATION:
1. Cover beets with vinegar.
2. Add cloves, sugar substitute, and lemon.
3. Separate onion slices into rings and add to beets.
4. Chill before serving.

BROCCOLI AND RICE CASSEROLE

Yield: 6 servings	**Each serving may be exchanged**
Each serving: ¾ cup	**for:** 1 Bread
	1 Meat
	1 Vegetable

INGREDIENTS:

1 (10-ounce) package frozen chopped broccoli

½ cup chopped onion

½ cup chopped celery

1 teaspoon reduced-calorie margarine

1 (10¾-ounce) can cream of chicken soup

1 cup grated low-fat process American cheese

1½ cups cooked rice

¼ teaspoon salt

⅛ teaspoon pepper

¼ teaspoon liquid pepper

1 tablespoon bread crumbs

STEPS IN PREPARATION:
1. Cook broccoli according to package directions; drain well.
2. Sauté onion and celery in margarine in nonstick skillet until clear.
3. Mix broccoli, soup, and cheese; add to celery and onion.
4. Stir in rice, salt, and peppers.
5. Put into nonstick 1½-quart casserole; top with bread crumbs.
6. Bake at 350° for 45 minutes, and serve.

Good sources of ascorbic acid (Vitamin C) are citrus fruits and juices, strawberries, cantaloupes, tomatoes, broccoli, green vegetables, cabbage, and potatoes.

BROCCOLI-CORN CASSEROLE

Yield: 8 servings **Each serving:** ⅓ cup	**Each serving may be exchanged** **for:** 1 Bread

INGREDIENTS:

1 (16-ounce) can cream-style
   corn
1 (10-ounce) package frozen
   chopped broccoli,
   cooked and drained
1 egg, beaten

12 saltine crackers, crushed
1 tablespoon minced onion
¼ teaspoon salt
⅛ teaspoon allspice
⅛ teaspoon pepper

STEPS IN PREPARATION:
1. Combine all ingredients; mix well.
2. Pour into nonstick 1-quart casserole.
3. Bake at 350° for 35 to 40 minutes, and serve.

GREEN BEAN CASSEROLE

Yield: 8 servings **Each serving:** ½ cup	**Each serving may be exchanged** **for:** ½ Medium-fat Meat 1 Vegetable

INGREDIENTS:

1 (10¾-ounce) package
   frozen chopped spinach,
   thawed
1 (9-ounce) package frozen
   green beans, thawed
½ cup chopped onion
¼ cup water
1 teaspoon salt
⅛ teaspoon garlic powder

1 teaspoon crushed dried
   basil
⅛ teaspoon nutmeg
⅛ teaspoon pepper
3 eggs, beaten
¼ cup grated low-fat process
   American cheese
Paprika

STEPS IN PREPARATION:
1. Drain spinach and green beans well.
2. Combine spinach, beans, onion, water, salt, garlic powder, basil, nutmeg, and pepper.
3. Cover and simmer for 10 minutes, stirring occasionally.
4. Remove from heat.
5. Gradually stir vegetable mixture into beaten eggs; stir mixture well.
6. Turn into 8-inch round baking dish.
7. Bake, uncovered, at 350° for about 20 minutes or until set.
8. Sprinkle with cheese and paprika.
9. Bake for 2 to 3 minutes more before serving.

SPANISH GREEN BEANS

Yield: 8 servings	**Each serving may be exchanged**
Each serving: ½ cup	**for:** 1 Vegetable

INGREDIENTS:

3¾ cups fresh green beans	½ teaspoon garlic powder
1 onion, chopped	¼ teaspoon pepper
2 tablespoons	5 medium tomatoes, diced
reduced-calorie	2 medium green peppers,
margarine	chopped
1½ teaspoons salt	

STEPS IN PREPARATION:
1. Cut beans into 1½-inch pieces; wash thoroughly, and drain.
2. Sauté onion in margarine in nonstick skillet until tender.
3. Add beans, salt, garlic powder, and pepper.
4. Cover and continue to cook over low heat for 10 minutes, stirring frequently.
5. Stir in tomatoes and green pepper.
6. Cover and simmer 25 to 30 minutes or until beans are tender.

MARINATED GREEN BEANS AND ONIONS

Yield: 4 servings **Each serving:** ½ cup	**Each serving may be substituted** **for:** 1 Vegetable ½ Fat

INGREDIENTS:

2 cups canned green beans, drained

1 cup reduced-calorie Italian salad dressing

1 small onion, sliced

¼ teaspoon salt

⅛ teaspoon pepper

STEPS IN PREPARATION:
1. Combine all ingredients in large bowl.
2. Mix well.
3. Refrigerate overnight.

Note: Mixture may be served hot or cold.

CARROTS IN "BUTTER" SAUCE

Yield: 10 servings **Each serving:** ⅓ cup	**Each serving may be exchanged** **for:** 1 Vegetable

INGREDIENTS:

3 cups sliced carrots

2 tablespoons reduced-calorie margarine

1 tablespoon all-purpose flour

1 cup fat-free chicken broth

¼ cup chopped green pepper

1 tablespoon dry butter substitute

½ teaspoon dried onion

½ teaspoon fresh parsley

STEPS IN PREPARATION:
1. Cook carrots, covered, in small amount of salted water until tender.
2. Drain and set aside.

3. Melt margarine in nonstick saucepan.
4. Add flour and stir until smooth.
5. Cook 1 minute, stirring constantly.
6. Gradually add broth; cook over medium heat, stirring constantly, until thickened.
7. Gently stir in carrots and remaining ingredients.
8. Heat well and serve.

"BUTTERY" GRATED CARROTS

Yield: 8 servings	**Each serving may be exchanged**
Each serving: ½ cup	**for:** 1 Vegetable

INGREDIENTS:

2 pounds carrots, peeled and grated (medium grate)
2 tablespoons water
1 tablespoon salad oil

½ teaspoon finely chopped garlic
½ teaspoon salt
⅛ teaspoon pepper
1 tablespoon dry butter substitute

STEPS IN PREPARATION:
1. Place carrots in skillet with tight-fitting lid.
2. Add water, salad oil, garlic, salt, and pepper.
3. Toss lightly.
4. Cover skillet and cook over medium heat 10 to 15 minutes or until tender, stirring occasionally.
5. Remove from heat.
6. Sprinkle butter substitute over mixture; blend and serve.

Cook vegetables in a small amount of water for short periods to keep vitamin destruction low.

CARROTS VICHY

Yield: 6 servings Each serving: ½ cup	Each serving may be exchanged for: 1 Vegetable

INGREDIENTS:

1 tablespoon reduced-calorie margarine
3 cups sliced carrots
¾ cup boiling water
1 teaspoon salt
¼ teaspoon nutmeg
⅛ teaspoon pepper

¼ cup chopped parsley
½ teaspoon monosodium glutamate
Sugar substitute to equal 2 teaspoons sugar
1 tablespoon lemon juice

STEPS IN PREPARATION:

1. Place margarine in saucepan.
2. Add carrots, boiling water, salt, nutmeg, and pepper.
3. Cover; simmer 8 to 10 minutes or until crisp-tender.
4. Stir in remaining ingredients, and serve.

CAULIFLOWER QUICHE

Yield: 8 servings Each serving: 1/8th quiche	Each serving may be exchanged for: ½ Bread 1 Medium-fat Meat

INGREDIENTS:

1⅔ cups cooked rice
2 cups cauliflower, chopped
1 cup skim milk
2 eggs, beaten
1 cup shredded low-fat process American cheese

½ teaspoon salt
Dash of pepper
Dash of nutmeg
¼ teaspoon liquid pepper

STEPS IN PREPARATION:

1. Gently press rice on bottom and sides of 9-inch nonstick pie pan.

2. Cook cauliflower in small amount of water 5 minutes or until crisp-tender.
3. Spoon over rice.
4. Mix remaining ingredients; pour over cauliflower.
5. Bake at 375° for 30 to 35 minutes.
6. Cut into 8 equal portions and serve.

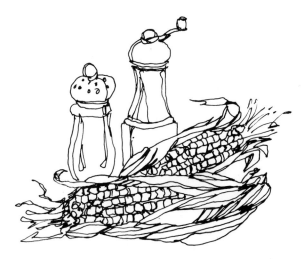

ROASTED CORN ON THE COB

Yield: 4 servings	Each serving may be exchanged
Each serving: ½ (4-inch) ear	for: 1 Bread

INGREDIENTS:

2 (8-inch) ears fresh corn	Dash of salt
4 teaspoons reduced-calorie margarine	Dash of pepper

STEPS IN PREPARATION:
1. Turn back corn husk and remove silk.
2. Spread ear with margarine; sprinkle with salt and pepper.
3. Pull husk back up, tying tightly.
4. Roast on grill over hot coals for 20 to 30 minutes; turn often.

FRESH "FRIED" CORN

Yield: 6 servings	Each serving may be exchanged
Each serving: ⅓ cup	for: 1 Bread

INGREDIENTS:

10 ears fresh corn or enough for 2 cups cut corn	⅛ teaspoon pepper (optional)
½ cup skim milk	1 tablespoon reduced-calorie
1 teaspoon salt	margarine

STEPS IN PREPARATION:

1. Shuck corn, and remove silk from ears.
2. Cut kernels from cob.
3. Scrape cobs gently with back of knife to get juice.
4. Stir milk, salt, and pepper, if desired, into corn.
5. Melt margarine in heavy skillet.
6. Pour corn mixture into skillet.
7. Simmer until tender, stirring often.

MEXICAN CORN

Yield: 7 servings	Each serving may be exchanged
Each serving: ⅓ cup	for: 1 Bread

INGREDIENTS:

2 cups whole kernel corn, drained	1 teaspoon salt
¼ cup chopped green pepper	¼ teaspoon oregano
¼ cup chopped red pepper	¼ teaspoon allspice
½ cup diced onion	1 cup peeled and diced fresh tomato
2 tablespoons reduced-calorie margarine	

STEPS IN PREPARATION:
1. Combine all ingredients, except tomato, in large nonstick skillet.
2. Cover; cook over medium heat 7 minutes, stirring occasionally.
3. Add tomato.
4. Cook, uncovered, for 2 minutes or until tomato is heated thoroughly.

CORN CASSEROLE

Yield: 6 servings **Each serving:** ½ cup	**Each serving may be exchanged** **for:** 1½ Bread 1 Fat

INGREDIENTS:

3 cups whole kernel corn, drained
¼ cup skim milk
1 egg, separated
½ teaspoon salt

3 tablespoons reduced-calorie margarine
1 teaspoon vanilla extract
Sugar substitute to equal 1 tablespoon sugar

STEPS IN PREPARATION:
1. Combine corn, milk, egg yolk, salt, margarine, vanilla, and sugar substitute in medium mixing bowl; stir well.
2. Beat egg white until stiff but not dry; fold into corn mixture.
3. Spoon into nonstick 8-inch square baking dish.
4. Bake at 350° for 30 to 40 minutes or until set.

Plan your menus for the week, but stay flexible enough to substitute good buys when you spot them. By planning ahead, you can use leftovers in another day's meal.

CORN CUSTARD

Yield: 6 servings **Each serving:** ⅓ cup	**Each serving may be exchanged for:** 1 Bread ½ Fat

INGREDIENTS:

1 (16-ounce) can cream-style corn

2 eggs, slightly beaten

1 tablespoon chopped parsley

½ teaspoon onion salt

STEPS IN PREPARATION:
1. Combine all ingredients.
2. Pour into small nonstick casserole.
3. Set casserole in pan of warm water.
4. Bake at 325° for 1¼ hours or until set.

CORN PUDDING

Yield: 8 servings **Each serving:** ¼ cup	**Each serving may be exchanged for:** 1 Bread

INGREDIENTS:

2 cups whole kernel corn, drained

1 cup skim milk

2 eggs, well beaten

½ teaspoon salt

Sugar substitute to equal 1 teaspoon sugar

¼ teaspoon pepper

⅛ teaspoon allspice

STEPS IN PREPARATION:
1. Combine all ingredients.
2. Pour into small nonstick casserole.
3. Bake at 350° for 60 to 70 minutes or until knife comes out clean when inserted into center of pudding.

When reheating foods, warm quickly to retain as many vitamins as possible.

EGGPLANT CREOLE

Yield: 6 servings	**Each serving may be exchanged**
Each serving: ¼ cup	**for:** 1 Vegetable

INGREDIENTS:

1 small onion, chopped
1 small green pepper, chopped
1 (8-ounce) can tomato sauce
1 clove garlic, minced

½ teaspoon salt
¼ teaspoon oregano
⅛ teaspoon pepper
¼ teaspoon liquid pepper
1 small eggplant, peeled and diced

STEPS IN PREPARATION:

1. Combine all ingredients, except eggplant, in skillet.
2. Cover and cook over low heat 10 minutes.
3. Add eggplant; cover and cook 20 minutes, stirring occasionally.

OKRA CREOLE

Yield: 11 servings	**Each serving may be exchanged**
Each serving: ⅓ cup	**for:** ½ Bread

INGREDIENTS:

1 (16-ounce) can whole tomatoes, undrained
1½ cups sliced okra
1 (7-ounce) can whole kernel corn

½ cup chopped onion
½ cup chopped celery
½ teaspoon salt
¼ teaspoon pepper
⅛ teaspoon oregano

STEPS IN PREPARATION:

1. Coarsely chop tomatoes.
2. Combine all ingredients in heavy skillet.
3. Bring to a boil.
4. Reduce heat; cover and simmer 15 to 20 minutes or until okra is tender.

OKRA-TOMATO CASSEROLE

Yield: 8 servings
Each serving: ½ cup

**Each serving may be exchanged
for:** 1 Vegetable

INGREDIENTS:

6 cups sliced tender okra
3 medium fresh tomatoes,
    chopped
½ cup chopped onion
½ cup chopped green
    pepper

½ teaspoon salt
¼ teaspoon pepper
1 tablespoon dry butter
    substitute

STEPS IN PREPARATION:

1. Place layers of okra, tomatoes, onion, green pepper, salt, and pepper in nonstick 2½-quart casserole.
2. Repeat layers.
3. Top with dry butter substitute.
4. Bake at 350° for 1 hour.

HERBED NEW POTATOES

Yield: 6 servings
Each serving: 1 potato

**Each serving may be exchanged
for:** 1 Bread

INGREDIENTS:

6 small (2-inch diameter)
    new potatoes, unpeeled
1 tablespoon minced fresh
    parsley

¼ teaspoon salt
Dash of pepper
2 teaspoons reduced-calorie
    margarine

STEPS IN PREPARATION:

1. Cook potatoes, covered, in boiling water 20 minutes or until tender.
2. Drain and peel.
3. Combine remaining ingredients.
4. Toss each potato in parsley mixture, and serve.

HASH BROWN POTATOES

Yield: 4 servings	Each serving may be exchanged
Each serving: ½ cup	for: 1 Bread

INGREDIENTS:

2 cups raw potatoes,
   chopped or diced
½ teaspoon salt

¼ teaspoon pepper
¼ cup green onion
   (optional)

STEPS IN PREPARATION:

1. Place potatoes, salt, and pepper in nonstick skillet; cook approximately 2 minutes, stirring constantly.
2. Reduce heat, and add onions, if desired; cook potatoes about 30 minutes or until tender.
3. Spray occasionally with nonstick spray if necessary to keep potatoes from sticking to skillet.
4. Fold like an omelet, and serve.

POTATO CASSEROLE

Yield: 8 servings	Each serving may be exchanged
Each serving: ½ cup	for: 1 Bread

INGREDIENTS:

4 medium white potatoes,
   peeled and sliced
1 (10¾-ounce) can cream of
   mushroom soup
2 tablespoons chopped
   green pepper

2 tablespoons minced onion
½ teaspoon salt
⅛ teaspoon pepper
   (optional)

STEPS IN PREPARATION:

1. Combine all ingredients.
2. Place in nonstick 1-quart casserole.
3. Bake at 350° for 1 to 1½ hours or until potatoes are tender.

SPICED SWEET POTATOES

Yield: 6 servings	**Each serving may be exchanged**
Each serving: ¼ cup	**for:** 1 Bread
	½ Fat

INGREDIENTS:

2 cups sliced sweet	¼ teaspoon salt
potatoes, cooked or	¼ teaspoon cinnamon
canned	¼ teaspoon nutmeg
Brown sugar substitute to	3 tablespoons
equal 3 tablespoons	reduced-calorie
brown sugar	margarine

STEPS IN PREPARATION:
1. Arrange sweet potatoes in nonstick casserole.
2. Combine sugar substitute, salt, cinnamon, and nutmeg; sprinkle over sweet potatoes.
3. Dot with margarine.
4. Bake at 350° for 10 to 15 minutes, and serve.

DILLY SQUASH

Yield: 4 servings	**Each serving may be exchanged**
Each serving: ½ cup	**for:** 1 Vegetable

INGREDIENTS:

3 cups sliced yellow summer	1 tablespoon chopped fresh
squash	parsley
1 teaspoon minced onion	¼ teaspoon dried dill weed
½ teaspoon salt	1 tablespoon dry butter
¼ cup water	substitute

STEPS IN PREPARATION:
1. Steam squash, onion, and salt until tender in ¼ cup water.
2. Remove from heat and mash squash mixture.
3. Add parsley and dill weed; toss lightly.
4. Sprinkle with dry butter substitute and serve.

BAKED ZUCCHINI SQUASH

Yield: 4 servings	Each serving may be exchanged
Each serving: 2 squash halves	for: 1 Vegetable

INGREDIENTS:

4 small fresh zucchini, cut in half lengthwise
3 tablespoons minced onion
3 tablespoons chopped green pepper
¼ teaspoon salt
Sugar substitute to equal 2 teaspoons sugar

⅛ teaspoon allspice
⅛ teaspoon pepper
¼ cup plain low-fat yogurt
4 saltine crackers, crushed
1 tablespoon dry butter substitute

STEPS IN PREPARATION:

1. Place cut zucchini in saucepan; add just enough water to cover.
2. Boil 5 minutes or until barely tender.
3. Drain and cool.
4. Scoop out squash pulp and place in bowl, reserving squash hulls.
5. Combine squash pulp, onion, green pepper, salt, sugar substitute, allspice, pepper, and yogurt.
6. Spoon mixture into squash hulls.
7. Sprinkle with cracker crumbs and dry butter substitute.
8. Bake at 350° for 30 minutes.

Milk and milk products are the best source of calcium. Turnip and mustard greens, collards, kale, broccoli, and cabbage also furnish calcium.

SAUTÉED ZUCCHINI

Yield: 6 servings	**Each serving may be exchanged**
Each serving: ½ cup	**for:** 1 Vegetable

INGREDIENTS:

½ cup chopped onion
1 tablespoon reduced-calorie margarine
3½ cups sliced zucchini
1 cup sliced mushrooms

½ teaspoon salt
½ teaspoon thyme
¼ teaspoon pepper
¼ cup grated low-fat process American cheese

STEPS IN PREPARATION:

1. Sauté onion in margarine in nonstick skillet until tender.
2. Add sliced zucchini, mushrooms, salt, thyme, and pepper.
3. Cook over low heat, stirring often, 5 to 7 minutes or until zucchini is crisp-tender.
4. Sprinkle with cheese, and serve.

BAKED TOMATOES

Yield: 4 servings	**Each serving may be exchanged**
Each serving: 2 tomato halves	**for:** 1 Vegetable

INGREDIENTS:

4 medium tomatoes, cut in half
¼ teaspoon salt
⅛ teaspoon pepper
¼ cup breadcrumbs, toasted
3 tablespoons minced fresh parsley

⅛ teaspoon garlic powder
¼ teaspoon thyme
¼ teaspoon oregano
Fresh parsley sprigs for garnish (optional)

STEPS IN PREPARATION:

1. Place tomato halves, cut surface up, in 12- x 8- x 2-inch nonstick baking dish.

2. Sprinkle with salt and pepper.
3. Combine breadcrumbs, minced parsley, garlic powder, thyme, and oregano.
4. Mix well; spoon over each tomato half.
5. Bake at 350° for 12 to 15 minutes.
6. Garnish with parsley sprigs, if desired, and serve.

SCALLOPED TOMATOES

Yield: 8 servings	**Each serving may be exchanged**
Each serving: ½ cup	**for:** 1 Vegetable

INGREDIENTS:

1 (20-ounce) can tomatoes
1 beef bouillon cube
1 cup bread cubes
2 tablespoons chopped onion
2 tablespoons chopped celery
½ teaspoon salt
2 tablespoons dry butter substitute

STEPS IN PREPARATION:

1. Drain tomatoes, reserving liquid.
2. Heat liquid to boiling; add bouillon cube, stirring to dissolve.
3. Add tomatoes, bread cubes, onion, celery, and salt to liquid.
4. Sprinkle with dry butter substitute.
5. Pour into nonstick 1-quart casserole.
6. Bake at 400° for 25 minutes.

Wash or chop vegetables and open cans before you begin preparing any recipe. It is also a good idea to have most ingredients measured before beginning to cook.

STEWED TOMATOES

Yield: 6 servings	Each serving may be exchanged
Each serving: ½ cup	for: 1 Vegetable

INGREDIENTS:

3 cups canned tomatoes
2 slices bread, cubed
¼ teaspoon salt
⅛ teaspoon pepper
1 tablespoon reduced-calorie
   margarine

1 tablespoon chopped green
   pepper, (optional)*
1 tablespoon chopped
   onion, (optional)*

STEPS IN PREPARATION:
1. Combine all ingredients in pan.
2. Heat to serving temperature, and serve.

*Note: If green pepper and onion are used, sauté in the margarine until tender, and add to tomato mixture.

TURNIP GREENS

Yield: 5 servings	Each serving may be exchanged
Each serving: ½ cup	for: 1 Vegetable

INGREDIENTS:

2 pounds fresh turnip greens
3 cups water
½ teaspoon salt
½ cup chopped onion
2 teaspoons reduced-calorie
   margarine

⅛ teaspoon allspice
1 tablespoon all-purpose
   flour
Sugar substitute to equal 1
   teaspoon sugar
2 tablespoons vinegar

STEPS IN PREPARATION:
1. Combine greens, water, and salt in large Dutch oven.
2. Bring to a boil.
3. Reduce heat; simmer 1 hour or until tender.
4. Drain greens, reserving 1 cup liquid; set aside.

5. Sauté onion in margarine in nonstick skillet.
6. Add onion and allspice to drained greens.
7. Dissolve flour and sugar substitute in vinegar; add to reserved 1 cup liquid.
8. Add mixture to greens.
9. Cook over medium heat, stirring occasionally, until thickened.

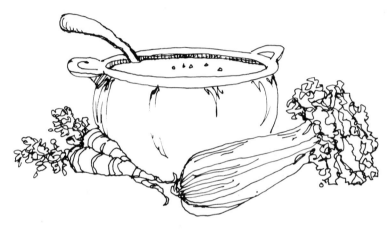

VEGETABLE SOUP

Yield: 8 servings	**Each serving may be exchanged**
Each serving: 1 cup	**for:** 2 Vegetable

INGREDIENTS:

1 beef bouillon cube	½ onion, sliced
1 cup boiling water	2 cups water
1½ cups potatoes, diced	2 cups canned tomatoes
½ cup carrots, diced	1 cup canned green peas
½ cup celery, diced	Dash of pepper

STEPS IN PREPARATION:

1. Dissolve bouillon cube in boiling water.
2. Add potatoes, carrots, celery, onion, and 2 cups water.
3. Cook until vegetables are tender.
4. Add tomatoes, peas, and pepper.
5. Simmer 10 minutes, and serve.

FREE FOODS AND BASICS

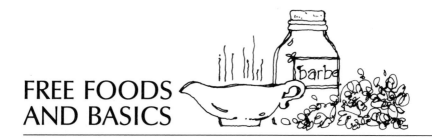

Americans are inclined to add many flavorings, spices, and other items to foods to bring out flavor and make them more palatable. Although many of these additives have little nutritive value, they enhance the taste and smell of food enabling people to enjoy it more. A few additives such as catsup, which has a tomato base and added sugar, add calories. Chili sauce is similar in caloric value to catsup.

Some food items can be considered basic because after certain ingredients are added, they result in a different product. An example is white sauce. Cheese may be added for variety and increased nutrient content. This section contains recipes for some of these basic foods.

Also included in this section are recipes for foods that can be considered "free," because they add very small amounts of carbohydrate, protein, and fat to the diet when eaten in the suggested amounts. See the Exchange List, page 17, for additional free items.

WHITE SAUCE

Yield: 1 cup	**Free food**
Each serving: 2 tablespoons	(1 serving per day)

INGREDIENTS:

1 tablespoon reduced-calorie margarine	1 cup skim milk
1 tablespoon all-purpose flour	½ teaspoon salt

STEPS IN PREPARATION:
1. Melt margarine in saucepan.
2. Blend in flour slowly.
3. Remove from heat.
4. Add milk, stirring constantly.
5. Return to low heat, and stir slowly but steadily until sauce boils.
6. Add salt.
7. Remove from heat.

Note: Sauce may be served over diced meats such as ham, chicken, or tuna or over vegetables such as green peas or white potatoes, or over hard-cooked eggs.

CHEESE SAUCE

Yield: 1 cup	**Each serving may be exchanged**
Each serving: ¼ cup	**for:** ½ Non-fat milk

INGREDIENTS:

1 cup white sauce	½ cup grated low-fat process American cheese

STEPS IN PREPARATION:
1. Make white sauce as directed above.
2. Add grated cheese.
3. Continue stirring until cheese melts; don't overcook.

Note: This sauce may be served over vegetables such as broccoli, asparagus, or cauliflower.

FAT-FREE CHICKEN "CREAM" GRAVY

Yield: 1 cup	**Free Food**
Each serving: 2 tablespoons	(Up to 2 servings per day)

INGREDIENTS:

2 tablespoons flour
¼ cup skim milk
1 cup fat-free chicken broth
  or fat-free drippings

½ teaspoon dried minced
  onion
Salt and pepper to taste

STEPS IN PREPARATION:
1. Add flour to skim milk; beat or stir until smooth.
2. Place broth or drippings and onion in saucepan; heat to boiling.
3. Add flour-milk mixture to broth very slowly, stirring constantly; season to taste.
4. Reduce heat; cook 5 minutes, stirring constantly.

FAT-FREE GRAVY

Yield: 3 cups	**Free food**
Each serving: 2 tablespoons	(Up to 2 servings per day)

INGREDIENTS:

2 tablespoons cornstarch or
  arrowroot
2 cups fat-free meat
  drippings*, broth or
  bouillon, divided
¼ teaspoon salt
¼ teaspoon pepper

½ cup minced onion
  (optional)
½ cup chopped mushrooms
  (optional)
2 tablespoons minced
  parsley (optional)

STEPS IN PREPARATION:
1. Add cornstarch or arrowroot to ½ cup fat-free meat drippings, broth, or bouillon and mix well.
2. Heat remaining liquid in saucepan.
3. Add cornstarch mixture to heating liquid.

4. Add salt, pepper and, if desired, optional ingredients.
5. Simmer until mixture thickens, stirring constantly.

*Note: To make fat-free meat drippings, refrigerate juices from cooked meats, skim the fat off top of juices, and discard. Use the fat-free juices for gravy or seasoning vegetables.

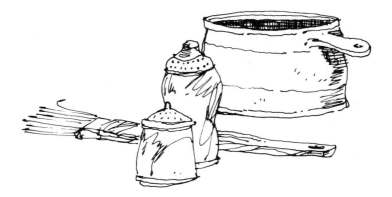

BARBECUE SAUCE

Yield: 1¼ cups	**Free food**
Each serving: 2 tablespoons	(Up to 2 servings per day)

INGREDIENTS:

½ cup lemon juice
⅓ cup cider vinegar
¼ cup cold water
¼ cup tomato juice
½ teaspoon salt
½ teaspoon onion powder
⅛ teaspoon garlic powder
Sugar substitute to equal 4
    teaspoons sugar

1 teaspoon dry mustard
½ teaspoon paprika
½ teaspoon pepper
½ teaspoon red pepper
⅛ teaspoon oregano
1 teaspoon liquid pepper

STEPS IN PREPARATION:

1. Combine ingredients in saucepan.
2. Heat to boiling.
3. Cool and refrigerate until served.

COCKTAIL SAUCE

Yield: ½ cup	Free food
Each serving: 2 tablespoons	(Up to 2 servings per day)

INGREDIENTS:

½ cup tomato sauce
1 teaspoon finely chopped parsley
½ teaspoon salt
Sugar substitute to equal 2 teaspoons sugar

Dash of onion powder
⅛ teaspoon oregano
1 teaspoon lemon juice
½ teaspoon Worcestershire sauce
½ teaspoon horseradish

STEPS IN PREPARATION:

1. Combine all ingredients; mix well.
2. Refrigerate until served.

CRANBERRY SAUCE

Yield: 3¾ cups	Free food
Each serving: 2 tablespoons	(Up to 3 servings per day)

INGREDIENTS:

½ cup water
2 tablespoons grated orange rind
Sugar substitute to equal 1 cup sugar

¼ teaspoon salt
⅛ teaspoon cinnamon
Dash of cloves
4 cups fresh ripe cranberries
½ teaspoon vanilla extract

STEPS IN PREPARATION:

1. Combine water, orange rind, sugar substitute, salt, cinnamon, and cloves in saucepan.
2. Bring to a boil; simmer 5 minutes, stirring occasionally.
3. Add cranberries; simmer until skins pop.
4. Remove from heat, and add vanilla.
5. Refrigerate until served.

BREAD AND BUTTER PICKLE CHIPS

Yield: 1 quart	Free food
Each serving: ¼ cup	(Up to 3 servings per day)

INGREDIENTS:

1 quart dill pickle chips	Sugar substitute to equal 1
1 cup vinegar	cup sugar
1 cup water	

STEPS IN PREPARATION:
1. Rinse dill pickles in cold water.
2. Place rinsed pickles in large jar, and cover with cold water.
3. Cover and place in refrigerator for 8 hours.
4. Drain pickles, and add vinegar, water, and sugar substitute.
5. Put back in refrigerator for at least 24 hours before serving.

TOMATO MADRILENE

Yield: 4 servings	Free food
Each serving: ½ cup	(Limit to 1 serving per day)

INGREDIENTS:

1 tablespoon unflavored	¼ teaspoon Worcestershire
gelatin	sauce
1 cup fat-free consommé,	4 green pepper slices
divided	4 lemon wedges
1 cup tomato juice cocktail	

STEPS IN PREPARATION:
1. Soften gelatin in ¼ cup consommé.
2. Heat remainder of consommé, and stir into gelatin mixture.
3. Add tomato juice cocktail and Worcestershire sauce.
4. Chill until set.
5. Beat lightly with fork.
6. Serve in soup cups garnished with green pepper slice and lemon wedge.

JELLIED CONSOMMÉ

Yield: 4 servings	**Free food**
Each serving: ½ cup	(Limit to 1 serving per day)

INGREDIENTS:

1 tablespoon unflavored
   gelatin
2 cups fat-free bouillon,
   soup stock, or
   consommé, divided

4 lemon slices
1 tablespoon minced parsley

STEPS IN PREPARATION:

1. Soften gelatin in ¼ cup fat-free liquid.
2. Heat remainder of liquid, and stir into gelatin mixture.
3. Chill until set.
4. Beat lightly with fork.
5. Serve in soup cups garnished with lemon slice dipped in parsley.

FRUIT GELATIN

Yield: 3 servings	**Free food**
Each serving: ½ cup	(Limit to 2 servings per day)

INGREDIENTS:

1 envelope unflavored
   gelatin
1 (12-ounce) can
   fruit-flavored diet drink,
   divided

⅛ teaspoon salt
1 teaspoon lemon juice
Vanilla, almond, or other
   flavoring extract, to taste
Sugar substitute, to taste

STEPS IN PREPARATION:

1. Soften gelatin in ½ cup diet drink.
2. Heat remaining diet drink to boiling.
3. Add gelatin mixture, and stir until dissolved.
4. Add remaining ingredients.
5. Chill until set.

STRAWBERRY WHIP

Yield: 8 servings	Free food
Each serving: ½ cup	(Limit to one serving per day)

INGREDIENTS:

½ cup diet strawberry
   carbonated soda
2 envelopes unflavored
   gelatin
2 cups fresh strawberries,
   washed and hulled

1¼ cups crushed ice
Strawberry-flavored extract,
   to taste
Sugar substitute, to taste

STEPS IN PREPARATION:

1. Heat strawberry soda in saucepan.
2. Pour hot diet soda, dry gelatin, and 1 cup of strawberries into blender; cover and blend 30 seconds.
3. Add crushed ice; blend 20 seconds longer.
4. Add remaining strawberries; blend about 3 seconds.
5. Add strawberry-flavored extract and sugar substitute as desired.
6. Pour into chilled serving bowl; chill 1 hour or until partially set.
7. Spoon into 8 serving dishes.

POPSICLES

Yield: 3	Free food
Each serving: 1 popsicle	

INGREDIENTS:

1 (12-ounce) diet soda
3 (5-ounce) paper cups

3 wooden stir sticks

STEPS IN PREPARATION:

1. Pour soda into cups.
2. Freeze until slightly set; add sticks.
3. Freeze until hard.
4. Peel away cup before serving.

WHIPPED TOPPING

Yield: ½ cup	**Each serving may be exchanged**
Each serving: ¼ cup	**for:** ½ Non-fat Milk

INGREDIENTS:
¼ cup cold water
¼ cup powdered skim milk

Sugar substitute to equal 2
 tablespoons sugar
½ teaspoon lemon juice

STEPS IN PREPARATION:
1. Chill bowl and beaters.
2. Combine water and powdered skim milk; beat until mixture begins to stiffen.
3. Add sugar substitute and lemon juice.
4. Continue to beat until stiff.

Note: Serve on fruits, gelatin, or other desserts.

FRESH STRAWBERRY SPREAD

Yield: 17 servings	**Free food**
Each serving: 1 tablespoon	(Up to 2 servings per day)

INGREDIENTS:
1 pint fresh ripe
 strawberries, washed and
 hulled
1 tablespoon cold water
1 tablespoon lemon juice
1 teaspoon dry unflavored
 gelatin

2 tablespoons cold water
Sugar substitute to equal 2
 tablespoons sugar
½ teaspoon vanilla

STEPS IN PREPARATION:
1. Cut strawberries into small pieces.
2. Place in heavy saucepan with 1 tablespoon cold water and lemon juice.
3. Partially crush berries.
4. Bring to boil; stir and cook rapidly about 5 minutes or until berries are cooked.

5. Meanwhile, soak gelatin in 2 tablespoons water.
6. Remove berries from heat.
7. Add gelatin, sugar substitute, and vanilla to berry mixture; stir to blend well.
8. Pour into hot (12- to 16-ounce) jar.
9. Cover lightly until cooled.
10. Cover tightly and store in refrigerator.

Note: May be used as a spread on bread, toast, muffins, crackers, etc.

APPLE JELLY

Yield: 22 servings	**Free food**
Each serving: 1 tablespoon	(Up to 2 servings per day)

INGREDIENTS:

1½ cups unsweetened apple juice
¾ teaspoon lemon juice
6 whole cloves
1 stick cinnamon
1½ teaspoons unflavored gelatin
⅓ cup cold water
Sugar substitute to equal ½ cup sugar

STEPS IN PREPARATION:
1. Combine juices, cloves, and cinnamon in heavy saucepan.
2. Bring to a boil, and simmer 10 minutes.
3. Meanwhile, soak gelatin in cold water.
4. Remove juice from heat; discard cloves and cinnamon.
5. Add gelatin and sugar substitute; mix well to dissolve.
6. Pour carefully into two hot, clean half-pint jars.
7. Cover lightly until cooled.
8. Cover tightly and store in refrigerator.

Note: Use as a spread on bread, toast, crackers, etc.

Read nutrition labels to determine your best buy.

Nutrient Chart

NUTRIENT	FUNCTIONS IN YOUR BODY	MAJOR FOOD SOURCES
Carbohydrates	Supply energy. Help body use other nutrients.	Cereals, fruits, vegetables, breads, sugars, milk, honey, cakes, cookies, pies, pasta.
Fats	Supply energy. Help maintain body temperature. Transport fat-soluble vitamins.	Margarine, butter, oils, shortening, cream, nuts, bacon, olives, whole milk.
Proteins	Build and repair body tissues. Help balance body chemicals. Supply energy.	Meat, poultry, fish, milk, cheese, nuts, dried peas and beans.
Vitamins		
Vitamin A	Helps eyes adjust to dim light. Helps keep skin healthy. Helps resist infection. Helps bones grow.	Liver, butter, cream, whole milk, egg yolk, broccoli, collards, spinach, carrots, sweet potatoes, pumpkin, winter squash, apricots, cantaloupe, greens.
Vitamin C	Helps hold body cells together. Helps heal wounds. Helps build bones and teeth. Helps absorb iron.	Oranges, grapefruit, cantaloupe, strawberries, raw cabbage, tomatoes, broccoli, green pepper.
Vitamin D	Helps body use calcium and phosphorous.	Liver, fortified milk, egg yolk (exposure to sunlight produces vitamin D in the skin).
Vitamin E	Helps keep red blood cells intact. Helps keep body fats intact.	Wheat germ, polyunsaturated vegetable oils.

Vitamin K	Is necessary for clotting blood.	Liver, spinach, greens, cabbage, cauliflower.
Thiamin (B1)	Helps body get energy from food. Helps keep nervous system healthy. Promotes good appetite and digestion.	Liver and other organ meats, meats, especially pork, poultry, whole-grain and enriched breads and cereals, nuts, dried peas and beans.
Riboflavin (B2)	Helps body get energy from food. Promotes healthy skin, eyes, and clear vision.	Milk, organ meats, egg white, enriched breads and cereals.
Niacin	Helps body produce energy. Aids digestion and good appetite. Helps keep skin, tongue, nervous system, and digestive tract healthy.	Lean meat, fish, poultry, liver, peanuts, whole-grain and enriched breads and cereals.
Cobalamine (B12)	Helps build red blood cells. Promotes healthy nervous system.	Liver and other organ meats, meat, fish, poultry.
Pyridoxine (B6)	Helps body use food. Helps build blood cells.	Egg yolk, whole-grain cereals, liver, peanuts, soybeans.
Minerals		
Calcium	Builds bones and teeth. Helps clot blood. Helps nerves, muscles, and heart to function well.	Milk, cheese, yogurt, buttermilk, tofu.
Phosphorous	Builds bones and teeth. Helps body get energy from food.	Milk and milk products, meat, fish, poultry, eggs, nuts, dried peas and beans.

Nutrient Chart

NUTRIENT	FUNCTIONS IN YOUR BODY	MAJOR FOOD SOURCES
Minerals		
Iron	Forms part of red blood cells. Helps body get energy from food.	Liver and other organ meats, egg yolk, meat, poultry, oysters, enriched and whole-grain breads and cereals, dried peas and beans.
Sodium	Helps control water balance. Regulates nerve impulses and muscle contractions.	Salt, meat, fish, poultry, milk and milk products, eggs.
Potassium	Helps control water balance. Regulates nerve impulses, muscle contractions, and heart rhythm.	Fruits, vegetables, meat, fish, poultry, milk and milk products.
Iodine	Regulates energy.	Seafood, iodized salt.
Magnesium	Is part of bones and teeth. Helps body use carbohydrates. Helps regulate nerve and muscle contractions.	Whole-grain cereals, nuts, dried peas and beans, milk, meat, leafy green vegetables.
Copper	Helps form red blood cells. Aids absorption and use of iron. Helps body get energy from food.	Liver, shellfish, meat, nuts, dried peas and beans, whole-grain cereals.
Water	Helps build and bathe body cells. Aids digestion and absorption. Helps lubricate joints and organs. Regulates body temperature.	All liquids such as water, coffee, tea, soft drinks, fruit and vegetable juices, milk, ice.

Table of Equivalents for Sugar Substitutes

BRAND NAME	SUBSTITUTION FOR SUGAR	BRAND NAME	SUBSTITUTION FOR SUGAR
Adolph's (powder)		**Sucaryl (liquid)**	
2 shakes of jar	= 1 rounded teaspoon sugar	⅛ teaspoon	= 1 teaspoon sugar
¼ teaspoon	= 1 tablespoon sugar	⅓ teaspoon	= 1 tablespoon sugar
1 teaspoon	= ¼ cup sugar	½ teaspoon	= 4 teaspoons sugar
2½ teaspoons	= ⅔ cup sugar	1½ teaspoons	= ¼ cup sugar
1 tablespoon	= ¾ cup sugar	1 tablespoon	= ½ cup sugar
4 teaspoons	= 1 cup sugar		
		Superose (liquid)	
		4 drops	= 1 teaspoon sugar
Equal (powder)		⅛ teaspoon	= 2 teaspoons sugar
1 packet	= 2 teaspoons sugar	⅛ teaspoon plus 4 drops	= 1 tablespoon sugar
		1½ teaspoons	= ½ cup sugar
		1 tablespoon	= 1 cup sugar
Fasweet (liquid)		**Sugar Twin (powder)**	
⅛ teaspoon	= 1 teaspoon sugar	1 teaspoon	= 1 teaspoon sugar
¼ teaspoon	= 2 teaspoons sugar		
⅓ teaspoon	= 1 tablespoon sugar	**Sugar Twin, Brown (powder)**	
1 tablespoon	= ½ cup sugar	1 teaspoon	= 1 teaspoon brown sugar
2 tablespoons	= 1 cup sugar		

Sugar equivalents for various brand names of sugar substitutes are listed for your convenience only and not as an endorsement.

Table of Equivalents for Sugar Substitutes

BRAND NAME	SUBSTITUTION FOR SUGAR	BRAND NAME	SUBSTITUTION FOR SUGAR
Sweet N' Low (powder)		**Sweet Magic (powder)**	
1/10 teaspoon	= 1 teaspoon sugar	1 packet	= 2 teaspoons sugar
1 packet	= 2 teaspoons sugar		
1/3 teaspoon	= 1 tablespoon sugar		
1 teaspoon	= 1/4 cup sugar	**Sweet-10 (liquid)**	
1 1/4 teaspoons	= 1/3 cup sugar	10 drops	= 1 teaspoon sugar
2 teaspoons	= 1/2 cup sugar	1/2 teaspoon	= 4 teaspoons sugar
4 teaspoons	= 1 cup sugar	1 1/2 teaspoons	= 1/4 cup sugar
		1 tablespoon	= 1/2 cup sugar
Sweet N' Low, Brown (powder)		2 tablespoons	= 1 cup sugar
1/4 teaspoon	= 1 tablespoon brown sugar		
1 teaspoon	= 1/4 cup brown sugar	**Zero-Cal (liquid)**	
1 1/3 teaspoons	= 1/3 cup brown sugar	10 drops	= 1 teaspoon sugar
2 teaspoons	= 1/2 cup brown sugar	30 drops	= 1 tablespoon sugar
4 teaspoons	= 1 cup brown sugar	3/4 teaspoon	= 2 tablespoons sugar
		1 tablespoon	= 1/2 cup sugar
Sweet'ner (powder)		2 tablespoons	= 1 cup sugar
1 packet	= 2 teaspoons sugar		

Sugar equivalents for various brand names of sugar substitutes are listed for your convenience only and not as an endorsement.

Fast Food Exchanges*

PRODUCT	SERVING SIZE	EXCHANGES
ARBY'S		
Roast Beef Sandwich	1 (5 oz.)	2 Bread, 3 Medium-fat Meat
Beef & Cheese Sandwich	1 (6 oz.)	2½ Bread, 3 Medium-fat Meat, 1 Fat
Super Roast Beef Sandwich	1 (9.75 oz.)	4 Bread, 3 Medium-fat Meat, 2½ Fat
Junior Roast Beef Sandwich	1 (3 oz.)	1½ Bread, 1 Medium-fat Meat, 1 Fat
Ham & Cheese Sandwich	1 (5.5 oz.)	2 Bread, 3 Medium-fat Meat
Turkey Deluxe Sandwich	1 (8.5 oz.)	3 Bread, 3 Medium-fat Meat, 2 Fat
Club Sandwich	1 (9 oz.)	3 Bread, 3½ Medium-fat Meat, 2 Fat
Turkey Sandwich	1 (6 oz.)	2½ Bread, 2½ Medium-fat Meat, 1 Fat
Swiss King Sandwich	1 (9.75 oz.)	3½ Bread, 4 Medium-fat Meat, 3 Fat
BURGER KING		
Hamburger	1 (3.9 oz.)	2 Bread, 2 Medium-fat Meat
Cheeseburger	1 (4.4 oz.)	2 Bread, 2 Medium-fat Meat, 1 Fat
Double Cheeseburger	1 (6.3 oz.)	2 Bread, 4 Medium-fat Meat, 2 Fat
Whopper	1 (9.2 oz.)	3 Bread, 3 Medium-fat Meat, 4 Fat
Whopper with Cheese	1 (10.2 oz.)	3 Bread, 4 Medium-fat Meat, 5 Fat
Double Beef Whopper	1 (11.9 oz.)	3 Bread, 5½ Medium-fat Meat, 5 Fat
Double Beef Whopper with Cheese	1 (12.9 oz.)	3½ Bread, 6 Medium-fat Meat, 6 Fat
Whopper Jr.	1 (5.1 oz.)	2 Bread, 2 Medium-fat Meat, 2 Fat
Whopper Jr. with Cheese	1 (5.6 oz.)	2 Bread, 2 Medium-fat Meat, 3 Fat
French Fries	1 (2.4 oz.)	1½ Bread, 2 Fat
Onion Rings	1 (2.7 oz.)	2 Bread, 3 Fat

*Printed with permission from "Nutritive and Exchange Values for Fast Food Restaurants," Marion J. Franz, R.D., M.S., International Diabetes Center, Minneapolis, Minnesota, 1983.

Fast Food Exchanges*

PRODUCT	SERVING SIZE	EXCHANGES
CHURCH'S FRIED CHICKEN		
Chicken, Cooked/Boned, White	1 piece (100 grams)	½ Bread, 3 Medium-fat Meat, 1½ Fat
Chicken, Cooked/Boned, Dark	1 piece (100 grams)	½ Bread, 3 Medium-fat Meat, 1 Fat
HARDEE'S		
Hamburger	1 (3.8 oz.)	2 Bread, 2 Medium-fat Meat
Cheeseburger	1 (4 oz.)	2 Bread, 2 Medium-fat Meat, 1 Fat
Big Cheese	1 (5.9 oz.)	2 Bread, 4 Medium-fat Meat, 2 Fat
Big Deluxe	1 (8.8 oz.)	3 Bread, 4 Medium-fat Meat, 4 Fat
Big Twin	1 (5.7 oz.)	2 Bread, 3 Medium-fat Meat, 2 Fat
Roast Beef Sandwich	1 (5 oz.)	2½ Bread, 2 Medium-fat Meat, 1 Fat
Big Roast Beef	1 (5.8 oz.)	2 Bread, 3 Medium-fat Meat, 1 Fat
Hot Dog	1 (4.2 oz.)	2 Bread, 1 Medium-fat Meat, 3 Fat
Hot Ham & Cheese	1 (5 oz.)	2½ Bread, 2½ Medium-fat Meat
Big Fish Sandwich	1 (6.8 oz)	3 Bread, 2 Medium-fat Meat, 3 Fat
Chicken Fillet	1 (6.7 oz.)	3 Bread, 3 Medium-fat Meat, 2 Fat
Biscuit	1 (2.8 oz.)	2 Bread, 3 Fat
Sausage Biscuit	1 (3.9 oz.)	2 Bread, 1 Medium-fat Meat, 4 Fat
Sausage Biscuit with Egg	1 (5.6 oz.)	2 Bread, 2 Medium-fat Meat, 5 Fat
Steak Biscuit	1 (4.7 oz.)	3 Bread, 1 Medium-fat Meat, 3 Fat
Steak Biscuit with Egg	1 (5.6 oz.)	3 Bread, 2 Medium-fat Meat, 4 Fat
Ham Biscuit	1 (3.8 oz.)	2½ Bread, 1 Medium-fat Meat, 2 Fat
Ham Biscuit with Egg	1 (6.4 oz.)	2½ Bread, 2 Medium-fat Meat, 3 Fat
One Fried Egg	1 (1.7 oz.)	1 Medium-fat Meat, 1 Fat
Biscuit with Egg	1 (5.5 oz.)	2 Bread, 1 Medium-fat Meat, 3 Fat
French Fries	Small (2.5 oz.)	2 Bread, 2 Fat
French Fries	Large (4 oz.)	3 Bread, 4 Fat

KENTUCKY FRIED CHICKEN
Original Recipe Chicken
(Edible Portion)

Wing	1 (1.5 oz.)	1½ Medium-fat Meat
Drumstick	1 (1.6 oz.)	2 Lean Meat
Side Breast	1 (2.4 oz.)	½ Bread, 2 Medium-fat Meat
Thigh	1 (3 oz.)	½ Bread, 2½ Medium-fat Meat, 1 Fat
Keel	1 (3.3 oz.)	½ Bread, 3 Medium-fat Meat

Extra Crispy Chicken
(Edible Portion)

Wing	1 (1.8 oz.)	½ Bread, 1 Medium-fat Meat, 2 Fat
Drumstick	1 (2 oz.)	2 Medium-fat Meat
Side Breast	1 (2.9 oz.)	1 Bread, 2 Medium-fat Meat, 1½ Fat
Thigh	1 (3.7 oz.)	1 Bread, 2½ Medium-fat Meat, 2 Fat
Keel	1 (3.6 oz.)	1 Bread, 3 Medium-fat Meat

Mashed Potatoes	1 Order (3 oz.)	1 Bread
Gravy	1 Tbsp. (.5 oz.)	½ Fat
Roll	1 (.7 oz.)	1 Bread
Corn	1 (5½" Pc.)	2 Bread, ½ Fat
Cole Slaw	1 Order (¾ cup)	1 Bread, 1 Fat

Original Recipe Chicken Dinner—2 Pieces of Chicken, Mashed Potatoes, Gravy, Cole Slaw, Roll

Wing & Side Breast	11.2 oz.	3 Bread, 3½ Medium-fat Meat, 3 Fat
Drumstick & Thigh	12 oz.	3 Bread, 4 Medium-fat Meat, 3 Fat
Wing & Thigh	11.9 oz.	3 Bread, 4 Medium-fat Meat, 3 Fat

Fast Food Exchanges*

PRODUCT	SERVING SIZE	EXCHANGES
KENTUCKY FRIED CHICKEN (continued)		
Extra Crispy Chicken Dinner—2 Pieces of Chicken, Mashed Potatoes, Gravy, Cole Slaw, Roll		
Wing & Side	12 oz.	4 Bread, 3½ Medium-fat Meat, 5 Fat
Drumstick & Thigh	13 oz.	4 Bread, 4 Medium-fat Meat, 6 Fat
Wing & Thigh	12.9 oz.	4 Bread, 4 Medium-fat Meat, 6 Fat
Chicken Breast Sandwich	1 (5.5 oz.)	2 Bread, 3 Medium-fat Meat, 1½ Fat
Kentucky Fries	1 Order (3.4 oz.)	2 Bread, 1 Fat
McDONALD'S		
Hamburger	1 (3.5 oz.)	2 Bread, 1 Medium-fat Meat, 1 Fat
Cheeseburger	1 (4 oz.)	2 Bread, 1½ Medium-fat Meat, 1 Fat
Quarter Pounder	1 (5.8 oz.)	2 Bread, 3 Medium-fat Meat, 1 Fat
Quarter Pounder with Cheese	1 (6.7 oz.)	2 Bread, 4 Medium-fat Meat, 2 Fat
Big Mac	1 (7 oz.)	3 Bread, 3 Medium-fat Meat, 3 Fat
Filet-O-Fish	1 (4.8 oz.)	2½ Bread, 1 Medium-fat Meat, 4 Fat
McChicken Sandwich	1	3 Bread, 2 Medium-fat Meat, 2 Fat
Chicken McNuggets	1 Order	1 Bread, 3 Medium-fat Meat, 1 Fat
Ham Biscuit	1	3 Bread, 2 Medium-fat Meat, 2 Fat
Sausage Biscuit	1	3 Bread, 2 Medium-fat Meat, 6 Fat
McFeast	1	2 Bread, 3 Medium-fat Meat, 3 Fat
McRib	1 Order	3 Bread, 3 Medium-fat Meat, 1 Fat
French Fries	1 Reg. Bag (2.4 oz.)	2 Bread, 2 Fat
Egg McMuffin	1 (4.8 oz.)	2 Bread, 2 Medium-fat Meat, 1 Fat
Scrambled Eggs	1 Order (3.4 oz.)	2 Medium-fat Meat, 1 Fat
Sausage Patties	1 Order (1.8 oz.)	1 Medium-fat Meat, 3 Fat

English Muffin with Butter	1 Whole (2 oz.)	2 Bread, 1 Fat
Hash Brown Potatoes	1 Order (2 oz.)	1 Bread, 1 Fat
Hot Mustard Sauce	1 Order	1 Fruit, ½ Fat
Barbecue Sauce	1 Order	1 Fruit
Sweet and Sour Sauce	1 Order	1½ Fruit

PIZZA HUT

Thin 'N Crispy Pizza

Beef	3 slices (½ 10" pizza)	3 Bread, 3 Medium-fat Meat, 1 Fat
Pork	3 slices (½ 10" pizza)	3 Bread, 3 Medium-fat Meat, 1½ Fat
Cheese	3 slices (½ 10" pizza)	3½ Bread, 3 Medium-fat Meat
Pepperoni	3 slices (½ 10" pizza)	3 Bread, 2½ Medium-fat Meat, 1 Fat
Supreme	3 slices (½ 10" pizza)	3 Bread, 3 Medium-fat Meat, 1 Fat

Thick 'N Chewy Pizza

Beef	3 slices (½ 10" pizza)	5 Bread, 4 Medium-fat Meat
Pork	3 slices (½ 10" pizza)	5 Bread, 4 Medium-fat Meat
Cheese	3 slices (½ 10" pizza)	5 Bread, 3 Medium-fat Meat
Pepperoni	3 slices (½ 10" pizza)	4½ Bread, 3 Medium-fat Meat
Supreme	3 slices (½ 10" pizza)	5 Bread, 4 Medium-fat Meat

TACO BELL

Bean Burrito	1 (5.8 oz.)	3 Bread, 1 Medium-fat Meat, 1 Fat
Beef Burrito	1 (6.5 oz.)	2½ Bread, 3 Medium-fat Meat, 1 Fat
Beef Tostada	1 (6.5 oz.)	1½ Bread, 2 Medium-fat Meat, 1 Fat
Bellbeefer	1 (4.3 oz.)	1½ Bread, 2 Medium-fat Meat, 1 Fat
Bellbeefer with Cheese	1 (4.8 oz.)	1½ Bread, 2 Medium-fat Meat
Burrito Supreme	1 (8 oz.)	3 Bread, 2 Medium-fat Meat, 2 Fat
Combination Burrito	1 (6 oz.)	3 Bread, 2 Medium-fat Meat, 1 Fat
Enchirito	1 (7 oz.)	3 Bread, 3 Medium-fat Meat, 1 Fat
Taco	1 (3 oz.)	1 Bread, 2 Medium-fat Meat
Tostada	1 (5 oz.)	1½ Bread, 1 Medium-fat Meat

Fast Food Exchanges*

PRODUCT	SERVING SIZE	EXCHANGES
WENDY'S		
Hamburger, Single	1 (7 oz.)	2 Bread, 3 Medium-fat Meat, 2 Fat
Hamburger, Double	1 (10 oz.)	2 Bread, 6 Medium-fat Meat, 2 Fat
Hamburger, Triple	1 (12.7 oz.)	2 Bread, 8½ Medium-fat Meat, 1 Fat
Cheeseburger, Single	1 (8.5 oz.)	2 Bread, 4 Medium-fat Meat, 3 Fat
Cheeseburger, Double	1 (11.5 oz.)	3 Bread, 6 Medium-fat Meat, 3 Fat
Cheeseburger, Triple	1 (14 oz.)	2 Bread, 10 Medium-fat Meat, 2 Fat
Chili	8.8 oz.	1½ Bread, 2 Lean Meat
French Fries	1 bag (4.2 oz.)	3 Bread, 3 Fat

Spice and Herb Chart

SPICE OR HERB	MEATS, FISH, AND POULTRY	VEGETABLES AND PASTA	SALADS	EGGS AND CHEESE
Basil	Lamb, Pork, Liver, Veal, Fish Fillets, Shrimp, Tuna, Chicken, Venison, Duck, Turkey	Peas, Eggplant, Green Beans, Cauliflower, Squash, Tomatoes, Onions, Soups	Egg, Seafood, Tossed Green, Tomato, Chicken, Cucumber	Scrambled Eggs, Cheese Strata, Omelets, Cheese Sauce
Bay Leaves	Stews, Pot Roast, Tripe, Fish, Tongue, Corned Beef	Beets, Carrots, Stewed Tomatoes, Boiled Potatoes, Soups	Aspic, Fish	
Black Pepper	Steaks, Chops, Roast, Stews, Chicken, Game, Casseroles	Green Beans, Squash, Beets, Spinach, Peas	Tossed Green, Potato, Pickled Beets, Bean	
Caraway	Pork, Tripe, Liver, Lamb Stew, Beef Stew, Tongue	Potatoes, Sauerkraut, Carrots, Cabbage, Noodles, Asparagus	Cole Slaw, Beets, Green Bean, Cucumber	
Cloves	Baked Ham, Stews, Pot Roast, Spiced Tongue, Game Stews, Venison, Roast Chicken	Winter Squash, Onions, Tomatoes, Sweet Potatoes	Spiced Apple, Spiced Peach	
Dill Weed	Corned Beef, Beef Stew, Pork Stew, Pork Roast, Fish, Chicken, Game Stews	Noodles, New Potatoes, Green Vegetables, Cauliflower	Tossed Green, Green Beans, Cucumber, Potato, Pickled Beet, Cole Slaw, Tuna	Deviled Eggs, Creamed Eggs, Cottage Cheese, Scrambled Eggs, Omelets

Spice and Herb Chart

SPICE OR HERB	MEATS, FISH, AND POULTRY	VEGETABLES AND PASTA	SALADS	EGGS AND CHEESE
Marjoram	Veal, Stews, Beef, Fish, Pork, Venison, Rabbit, Chicken, Goose, Duck, Turkey	Carrots, Zucchini, Peas, Spinach, Soups, Onions	Tossed Green, Chicken, Seafood	Omelets, Scrambled Eggs, Soufflés
Oregano	Ground Beef, Pork, Lamb, Meat Loaf, Chicken, Guinea Hen, Shrimp, Lobster, Liver	Tomatoes, Cabbage, Lentils, Broccoli, Soups, Onions	Tomato Aspic, Fish, Cucumber, Bean, Potato	Soufflés, Omelets, Cheese Sauce, Scrambled Eggs
Paprika	Beef, Stew, Fish, Lobster, Chicken, Fish Chowder, Casseroles	Potato, Corn, Rice, Casseroles, Noodles	Potato, Macaroni, Chicken, Tuna	Deviled Eggs, Creamed Eggs, Cheese Sauce, Cheese Strata
Red Pepper	Stews, Italian Dishes, Chicken, Seafood Creole, Fish, Casseroles	Casseroles	Seafood, Chicken, Turkey	Cheese Strata, Cheese Sauce, Omelets
Rosemary	Pork, Veal, Poultry, Beef, Fish, Wild Fowl, Capon, Duck, Rabbit, Venison, Lamb	Peas, Spinach, Cauliflower, Turnips, Soups	Fruit, Tomato, Cucumber	Deviled Eggs, Scrambled Eggs, Soufflés

	Meats	Vegetables	Salads	Eggs & Cheese
Sage	Cottage Cheese, Stews, Pork, Lamb, Goose, Turkey, Rabbit, Fish, Chicken, Duck	Lima Beans, Eggplant, Onions, Tomatoes, Soups, Carrots	Tomato, Tossed Green, Bean	Cottage Cheese, Creamed Eggs, Soufflés
Savory	Turkey, Hamburger, Pork, Veal, Stews, Meat Loaf, Chicken, Rabbit, Fish Fillets, Shrimp	Beans, Rice, Lentils, Sauerkraut, Soups	Mixed Green, Bean, Tomato	Deviled Eggs, Scrambled Eggs, Omelets
Tarragon	Veal, Steaks, Chops, Chicken, Duck, Pheasant, Cornish Hens, Seafood, Lamb	Cauliflower, Beans, Lentils, Rice, Peas, Soups	Salmon, Tuna, Tossed Green, Bean, Chicken, Egg	Deviled Eggs, Cottage Cheese, Omelets
Thyme	Fish Fillets, Lamb, Beef, Meat Loaf, Stews, Liver, Chicken, Venison, Scallops, Turkey	Beets, Onions, Carrots, Brussel Sprouts, Zucchini, Asparagus	Pickled Beets, Tomato, Aspic, Cole Slaw, Chicken	Deviled Eggs, Soufflés, Omelets, Cottage Cheese
White Pepper	Stew, Veal, Fish, Casseroles	Cauliflower, Cabbage, Rice, Asparagus, Potatoes	Salmon, Tomato, Tuna, Shrimp, Chicken, Turkey	Deviled Eggs, Cheese Sauce, Creamed Eggs, Cheese Strata

DIETETIC FOOD EXPLANATIONS

DIETETIC GELATIN - a gelatin dessert product which contains a sugar substitute as a sweetener instead of sugar; ½-cup serving contains approximately 8 calories.

DIETETIC JELLY, JAM, OR MARMALADE - spreads which contain a sugar substitute as a sweetener instead of sugar; one tablespoon contains approximately 7 to 30 calories instead of the 50 to 60 calories per tablespoon found in regular sweetened spreads.

DIET SODA - a beverage which is made with a sugar substitute instead of sugar; one serving contains approximately 2 calories or less.

DIETETIC SYRUP - syrup which contains a sugar substitute instead of sugar; one tablespoon contains approximately 9 calories.

DRY BUTTER SUBSTITUTE - a 100% natural butter flavored product which is derived from butter but contains 99% less cholesterol than butter and 94% fewer calories than butter or margarine. Water can be added to the powder to form a liquid butter substitute which contains approximately 6 calories per tablespoon of liquid.

LOW-FAT PROCESS CHEESE - cheese which has been specially processed and contains 2 grams of fat per ounce instead of 4 to 10 grams of fat per ounce found in regular cheeses.

LOW-FAT YOGURT - yogurt which is made from 1% or 2% fat milk rather than whole milk which contains 4% fat.

REDUCED-CALORIE MARGARINE - margarine which contains half the fat of regular margarine due to a decrease in fat content from 80% to 40%; one teaspoon contains approximately 15 calories.

REDUCED-CALORIE MAYONNAISE - mayonnaise which contains half the calories of regular mayonnaise because of a decrease in fat content from 80% to 40%; one tablespoon contains approximately 50 calories.

REDUCED-CALORIE SALAD DRESSING - salad dressing which contains 33% to 50% less fat than the regular salad dressing; one teaspoon contains approximately 11 calories.

REDUCED-CALORIE WHIPPED TOPPING - whipped topping which contains half the fat content of regular whipped topping due to the use of coconut or soybean oil with fillers instead of cream. Whipped toppings may also be lower in calories when sugar substitute is used instead of sugar and water is used in place of milk or cream.

SOFT MARGARINE - margarine which contains more unhydrogenated fat than regular margarine; one teaspoon contains approximately 33 calories.

VEGETABLE COOKING SPRAY - a cholesterol- and salt-free vegetable compound in spray form which is used to coat cookware with a nonstick surface; one spray of this compound contains less than 7 calories.

WHIPPED MARGARINE - margarine which contains one-third the volume of regular margarine; one teaspoon contains approximately 22 calories. One teaspoon of whipped margarine weighs approximately 10 grams compared to one teaspoon of regular margarine which weighs 14 grams.

GLOSSARY

CALORIE - a unit of heat that measures the amount of energy in food.

CARBOHYDRATE - a major nutrient found in sugars, breads, cereals, vegetables, fruit, and milk; provides 4 calories per gram weight.

CHOLESTEROL - a fat-like substance which is made in the liver and found in animal foods.

DIABETES MELLITUS - failure of body cells to use carbohydrate because of inadequate production or use of insulin.

DIETETIC FOODS - foods prepared for special diets, such as low-fat, low-sodium, sugar-free, calorie-reduced, low-cholesterol—not all are suitable for diabetics.

DIGESTION - the breakdown of foods in the digestive tract into simple substances the body can use for energy and nourishment.

"FREE" FOODS - foods which have few calories and carbohydrates and do not need to be counted as Exchanges.

ENRICHED FOODS - foods made from refined grains to which one or more nutrients have been added to increase the nutrient value.

FAT - a major nutrient found in meats, eggs, milk and milk products, oils, margarine, salad dressings, and nuts which provides 9 calories per gram weight.

FIBER - that part of foods which is not digested and adds bulk but not calories to the diet.

FOOD EXCHANGE - a group of foods which contain similar nutrients.

GLUCOSE - a simple sugar found in the blood which is made either by the digestion of food or from other carbohydrate and protein sources found in the body.

GRAM - a unit of weight in the metric system; one ounce equals 28.25 grams.

HYPERGLYCEMIA - high blood glucose (sugar) levels.

HYPOGLYCEMIA - low blood glucose (sugar) levels.

INSULIN - a hormone made by the pancreas which is needed by the body to use carbohydrate.

INSULIN REACTION - a rapid fall in blood glucose level due to the action of injected insulin.

MEAL PLAN - a guide used to show the number of Exchanges to eat at each meal.

MINERALS - a group of nutrients necessary for life found in small amounts in foods.

MONOUNSATURATED FAT - a neutral fat which does not increase or decrease serum (blood) cholesterol levels.

NUTRIENT - a substance necessary for life and found in food.

NUTRITION - the process by which the body uses food to nourish cells.

POLYUNSATURATED FAT - a fat found in plants which tends to lower serum (blood) cholesterol levels.

PROTEIN - a major nutrient which is essential for life and needed for building and repairing body cells and which is found in meats, eggs, milk and milk products. Proteins provide 4 calories per gram weight.

SATURATED FAT - a fat which tends to raise serum (blood) cholesterol levels and is usually found as solid fat.

STARCH - a complex form of carbohydrate which is changed to sugar during digestion.

VITAMIN - a nutrient necessary for life found in small amounts in foods.

RECIPE INDEX

SUBJECT INDEX

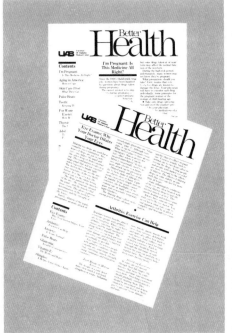
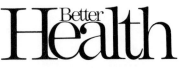